WORLD HEALTH ORGANIZATION

CORRIGENDA

ENVIRONMENTAL HEALTH CRITERIA
NO. 103

2-PROPANOL

Page 2, line 14:
Delete: 1.2-Propanol
Insert: 1.Alcohol, propyl

Page 2, line 15:
Delete: QV 223
Insert: QD 305.A4

This report contains the collective views of an international group of experts and does not necessarily represent the decisions or the stated policy of the United Nations Environment Programme, the International Labour Organisation, or the World Health Organization.

Environmental Health Criteria 103

2-PROPANOL

Published under the joint sponsorship of
the United Nations Environment Programme,
the International Labour Organisation,
and the World Health Organization

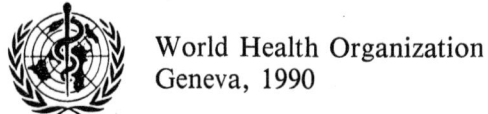

World Health Organization
Geneva, 1990

The International Programme on Chemical Safety (IPCS) is a joint venture of the United Nations Environment Programme, the International Labour Organisation, and the World Health Organization. The main objective of the IPCS is to carry out and disseminate evaluations of the effects of chemicals on human health and the quality of the environment. Supporting activities include the development of epidemiological, experimental laboratory, and risk-assessment methods that could produce internationally comparable results, and the development of manpower in the field of toxicology. Other activities carried out by the IPCS include the development of know-how for coping with chemical accidents, coordination of laboratory testing and epidemiological studies, and promotion of research on the mechanisms of the biological action of chemicals.

WHO Library Cataloguing in Publication Data

2-Propanol

(Environmental health criteria ; 103)

1.2-Propanol   I.Series

ISBN 92 4 157103 9   (NLM Classification: QV 223)
ISSN 0250-863X

© World Health Organization 1990

Publications of the World Health Organization enjoy copyright protection in accordance with the provisions of Protocol 2 of the Universal Copyright Convention. For rights of reproduction or translation of WHO publications, in part or *in toto*, application should be made to the Office of Publications, World Health Organization, Geneva, Switzerland. The World Health Organization welcomes such applications.

The designations employed and the presentation of the material in this publication do not imply the expression of any opinion whatsoever on the part of the Secretariat of the World Health Organization concerning the legal status of any country, territory, city or area or of its authorities, or concerning the delimitation of its frontiers or boundaries.

The mention of specific companies or of certain manufacturers' products does not imply that they are endorsed or recommended by the World Health Organization in preference to others of a similar nature that are not mentioned. Errors and omissions excepted, the names of proprietary products are distinguished by initial capital letters.

Computer typesetting by HEADS, Oxford OX7 2NY, England

PRINTED IN FINLAND
Vammalan Kirjapaino Oy
90/8460 — VAMMALA — 5000

CONTENTS

	Page
ENVIRONMENTAL HEALTH CRITERIA FOR 2-PROPANOL	10

1. SUMMARY 11

    1.1   Identity, physical and chemical properties, analytical methods 11
    1.2   Sources of human and environmental exposure . 11
    1.3   Environmental transport, distribution, and transformation 12
    1.4   Environmental levels and human exposure ... 12
    1.5   Kinetics and metabolism 13
    1.6   Effects on organisms in the environment 14
    1.7   Effects on experimental animals and *in vitro* test systems 14
    1.8   Health effects in human beings 16
    1.9   Summary of evaluation 18

2. IDENTITY, PHYSICAL AND CHEMICAL PROPERTIES, ANALYTICAL METHODS 20
    2.1   Identity 20
    2.2   Physical and chemical properties 21
    2.3   Analytical methods 22

3. SOURCES OF HUMAN AND ENVIRONMENTAL EXPOSURE 27
    3.1   Natural occurrence 27
    3.2   Man-made sources 27
            3.2.1   Production levels and processes 27
                    3.2.1.1 Production levels 27
                    3.2.1.2 Production processes 27
            3.2.2   Uses 28
            3.2.3   Waste disposal 30

	Page

4. ENVIRONMENTAL TRANSPORT, DISTRIBUTION,
   AND TRANSFORMATION 31

   4.1 Transport and distribution between media . . . 31
   4.2 Abiotic degradation 32
   4.3 Biotransformation 33
       4.3.1 Biodegradation 33
       4.3.2 Bioaccumulation 35

5. ENVIRONMENTAL LEVELS AND HUMAN
   EXPOSURE 36

   5.1 Environmental levels 36
   5.2 General population exposure 37
       5.2.1 Exposure via food 37
       5.2.2 Exposure via other consumer products 38
   5.3 Occupational exposure 40

6. KINETICS AND METABOLISM 44

   6.1 Absorption 44
       6.1.1 Animals 44
       6.1.2 Human beings 45
   6.2 Distribution 46
       6.2.1 Animals 46
       6.2.2 Human beings 46
   6.3 Metabolism 46
       6.3.1 Animals 46
       6.3.2 Human beings 48
   6.4 Elimination and excretion 50
       6.4.1 Animals 50
       6.4.2 Human beings 51

7. EFFECTS ON ORGANISMS IN THE
   ENVIRONMENT 52

   7.1 Aquatic organisms 52
   7.2 Terrestrial organisms 57

		Page
7.2.1	Microorganisms	57
7.2.2	Insects	57
7.2.3	Plants	57

8. EFFECTS ON EXPERIMENTAL ANIMALS AND *IN VITRO* TEST SYSTEMS 59

- 8.1 Single exposures 59
  - 8.1.1 Mortality 59
  - 8.1.2 Signs of intoxication 59
  - 8.1.3 Skin, eye, and respiratory tract irritation 61
- 8.2 Continuous or repeated exposures 62
- 8.3 Neurotoxicity and behavioural effects 64
- 8.4 Biochemical effects 66
  - 8.4.1 Effects on lipids in liver and blood ... 66
  - 8.4.2 Effects on microsomal enzymes 67
  - 8.4.3 Other biochemical findings 68
- 8.5 Immunological effects 68
- 8.6 Reproduction, embryotoxicity, and teratogenicity 69
- 8.7 Mutagenicity 70
- 8.8 Carcinogenicity 71
- 8.9 Factors modifying toxicity 72

9. EFFECTS ON MAN 73

- 9.1 General population exposure 73
  - 9.1.1 Poisoning incidents 73
  - 9.1.2 Controlled exposures 75
  - 9.1.3 Skin irritation; sensitization 76
- 9.2 Occupational exposure 77
  - 9.2.1 Epidemiology studies 77
  - 9.2.2 Interacting agents 79

		Page
10. EVALUATION OF HUMAN HEALTH RISKS AND EFFECTS ON THE ENVIRONMENT		80
10.1	Evaluation of human health risks	80
10.1.1	Exposure	80
10.1.2	Health effects	80
10.2	Evaluation of effects on the environment	82
11. RECOMMENDATIONS		84
12. PREVIOUS EVALUATIONS BY INTERNATIONAL BODIES		85
REFERENCES		86
RESUME		111
RESUMEN		123

WHO TASK GROUP MEETING ON ENVIRONMENTAL HEALTH CRITERIA FOR 2-PROPANOL

Members

Dr R. Drew, Department of Clinical Pharmacology, Flinders University of South Australia, Bedford Park, South Australia, Australia

Dr B. Gilbert, Company for Development of Technology Transfer (CODETEC), City University, Campinas, Brazil (*Rapporteur*)

Dr B. Hardin, Document Development Branch, Division of Standards Development and Technology Transfer, National Institute for Occupational Safety and Health, Cincinnati, Ohio, USA (*Chairman*)

Dr S.K. Kashyap, National Institute of Occupational Health, Ahmedabad, India

Professor M. Noweir, Occupational Health Research Centre, High Institute of Public Health, University of Alexandria, Alexandria, Egypt

Dr L. Rosenstein, Office of Toxic Substances, US Environmental Protection Agency, Washington, DC, USA

Professor I.V. Sanotsky, Chief, Department of Toxicology, Institute of Industrial Hygiene and Occupational Diseases, Moscow, USSR (*Vice-Chairman*)

Dr J. Sokal, Division of Industrial Toxicology, Institute of Occupational Medicine, Lodz, Poland

Dr H.J. Wiegand, Toxicology Department, Huls AG, Marl, Federal Republic of Germany

Dr K. Woodward, Department of Health, Medical Toxicology and Environmental Health Division, London, United Kingdom

Observers

    Dr K. Miller (Representing International Commission on Occupational Health (ICOH)), British Industrial Biological Research Association, Carshalton, Surrey, United Kingdom

Secretariat

    Professor F. Valić, Consultant, IPCS, World Health Organization, Geneva, Switzerland, *also* Vice-Rector, University of Zagreb, Zagreb, Yugoslavia (*Secretary*)

    Dr T. Vermeire, National Institute of Public Health and Environmental Hygiene, Bilthoven, Holland

Host Organization

    Dr S.D. Gangolli, British Industrial Biological Research Association, Carshalton, Surrey, United Kingdom

    Dr D. Anderson, British Industrial Biological Research Association, Carshalton, Surrey, United Kingdom

NOTE TO READERS OF THE CRITERIA DOCUMENTS

Every effort has been made to present information in the criteria documents as accurately as possible without unduly delaying their publication. In the interest of all users of the environmental health criteria documents, readers are kindly requested to communicate any errors that may have occurred to the Manager of the International Programme on Chemical Safety, World Health Organization, Geneva, Switzerland, in order that they may be included in corrigenda, which will appear in subsequent volumes.

* * *

A detailed data profile and a legal file can be obtained from the International Register of Potentially Toxic Chemicals, Palais des Nations, 1211 Geneva 10, Switzerland (Telephone no. 7988400/ 7985850).

ENVIRONMENTAL HEALTH CRITERIA FOR 2-PROPANOL

A WHO Task Group on Environmental Health Criteria for 2-Propanol met at the British Industrial Biological Research Association (BIBRA), Carshalton, Surrey, United Kingdom, from 10 to 14 April 1989. Dr S.D. Gangolli, who opened the meeting, welcomed the participants on behalf of the Department of Health, and Dr D. Anderson on behalf of BIBRA, the host institution. Dr F. Valić greeted the participants on behalf of the heads of the three IPCS cooperating organizations (UNEP/ILO/WHO). The Task Group reviewed and revised the draft criteria document and made an evaluation of the human health risks and effects on the environment of exposure to 1-propanol.

The drafts of this document were prepared by Dr T. VERMEIRE, National Institute of Public Health and Environmental Hygiene, Bilthoven, Netherlands. Dr F. VALIC was responsible for the overall scientific content of the document and Mrs M.O. HEAD of Oxford, England, for the editing.

The efforts of all who helped in the preparation and finalization of the document are gratefully acknowledged.

* * *

Partial financial support for the publication of this criteria document was kindly provided by the United States Department of Health and Human Services, through a contract from the National Institute of Environmental Health Sciences, Research Triangle Park, North Carolina, USA — a WHO Collaborating Centre for Environmental Health Effects. The United Kingdom Department of Health and Social Security generously supported the cost of printing.

1. SUMMARY

1.1 Identity, Physical and Chemical Properties, Analytical Methods

2-Propanol is a colourless highly flammable liquid with an odour resembling that of a mixture of ethanol and acetone. The compound is completely miscible with water, ethanol, acetone, chloroform, and benzene. Analytical methods are available for the detection of 2-propanol in various media (air, water, blood, serum, and urine) with detection limits for air, water, and blood of 2×10^{-5} mg/m^3, 0.04 mg/litre, and 1 mg/litre, respectively. Gas chromatographic methods (primarily using flame ionization detection) as well as paper electrophoresis and photoionization ion mobility spectrometry methods are available for the determination of 2-propanol in the various media.

1.2 Sources of Human and Environmental Exposure

World production of 2-propanol in 1975 was estimated to be more than 1100 kilotonnes and the global production capacity in 1984 was estimated to be more than 2000 kilotonnes. 2-Propanol is commonly manufactured from propene. The previously used strong acid and weak acid processes, which involved potentially hazardous intermediates and by-products, have now largely been replaced by the catalytic hydration process. The catalytic reduction of acetone is an alternative process.

2-Propanol has been identified as a metabolic product of a variety of microorganisms.

The compound has widespread solvent applications, and is used as a component of household and personal products including aerosol sprays, topically applied pharmaceutical products, and cosmetics. 2-Propanol is also used in the production of acetone and other chemicals, as a de-icing agent, as a preservative, in windscreen wiper concentrates, and as a flavour volatile in foodstuffs.

2-Propanol may enter the atmosphere, water, or soil following waste disposal and has been identified in the air and leachates from hazardous waste sites and landfills. It is emitted in waste gases and waste water from industrial sources, and may be removed from the latter by biological oxidation or reverse osmosis. Disperse airborne emissions will occur during the use of 2-propanol in consumer products.

1.3 Environmental Transport, Distribution, and Transformation

The main pathway of entry of 2-propanol into the environment is through its emission into the atmosphere during production, processing, storage, transport, use, and disposal. Emissions into soil and water also occur. The emissions to each environmental compartment are difficult to estimate. However, in 1976, the total release of this compound into the atmosphere was estimated to exceed 50% of the 2-propanol produced.

2-Propanol is rapidly removed from the atmosphere by reaction with hydroxyl radicals and by rain-out. The latter is responsible for the transport of 2-propanol from the atmosphere to soil or water. Once in the soil, it is likely to be very mobile and it increases soil permeability to some aromatic hydrocarbons. 2-Propanol is readily biodegradable, both aerobically and anaerobically.

It is not expected to bioaccumulate because it is biodegradable and is completely miscible in water, with a log n-octanol/water partition coefficient of 0.14 and a bioconcentration factor of 0.5.

1.4 Environmental Levels and Human Exposure

Exposure of the general population occurs through accidental or intentional ingestion, through the ingestion of food containing 2-propanol as a natural or added flavour volatile or as a solvent residue, and through inhalation during use. Concentrations have been found of between 0.2 and 325 mg/litre in non-alcoholic beverages and 50–3000 mg/kg in foods following the use of 2-propanol as a solvent in their production. Exposure of the general population through inhalation of ambient air is low, because of its rapid removal and degradation. Various sites have been monitored and time-weighted average concentrations of up to 35 mg/m^3 have been measured for urban sites.

Workers are exposed to 2-propanol during the production of the compound itself, and of acetone and other derivatives, and also during its use as a solvent. In the USA, it was estimated by the National Occupational Exposure Survey (1980–83) that over 1.8 million workers were potentially exposed. Concentrations of up to 1350 mg/m^3 have been measured at work-places, with time-weighted averages of up to about 500 mg/m^3.

1.5 Kinetics and Metabolism

2-Propanol is rapidly absorbed and distributed throughout the body after inhalation or ingestion. At high doses, gastrointestinal absorption is delayed. Blood levels of 2-propanol (detectable when ethanol is ingested simultaneously) or of its metabolite, acetone, are related to the exposure levels. Human volunteers who ingested a dose of 3.75 mg/kg (with 1200 mg ethanol/kg) in orange juice exhibited a peak level of 0.8 ± 0.3 mg free 2-propanol/litre in the blood, and 2.3 ± 1.4 mg/litre after incubation with aryl sulfatase, suggesting sulfation. Workers exposed to vapour (8–647 mg/m^3) showed concentrations of 3–270 mg/m^3 in the alveolar air but, in this case, acetone, not 2-propanol, was found in the blood and urine. In treated laboratory animals, 2-propanol was detected not only in the blood but also in the spinal fluid, liver, kidneys, and brain. It passes the blood–brain barrier twice as effectively as ethanol.

2-Propanol is excreted partly unchanged and partly as acetone, mainly via the lungs, but also via saliva and gastric juice. Reabsorption may follow excretion via the last 2 routes. The metabolism to acetone via liver alcohol dehydrogenase (ADH) is rather slow since the relative affinity of ADH for 2-propanol is lower than it is for ethanol. *In vitro*, human ADH with 2-propanol showed 9-10% of the activity of the enzyme with ethanol as substrate. *In vitro*, rat liver microsomal oxidases are also capable of oxidizing 2-propanol. In human beings, acetone is excreted unchanged, primarily via the lungs, and minimally by the kidneys. Acetone levels in alveolar air, blood, and urine increase with the extent and the duration of exposure to 2-propanol. The elimination of

2-propanol and acetone from the body is first order, and half-lives in human beings are 2.5–6.4 h and 22 h, respectively.

1.6 Effects on Organisms in the Environment

The toxicity of 2-propanol for aquatic organisms, insects, and plants is low. The inhibitory threshold for cell multiplication of a sensitive protozoan species ranged from 104 to 4930 mg/litre under various experimental conditions. Progressing higher through the phylogenetic chain, various species of crustacea, including *Daphnia magna,* showed EC_{50}s at levels ranging from 2285 to 9714 mg/litre. LC_{50}s (96-h) for freshwater fish ranged from 4200 to 11 130 mg/litre. Data obtained for fruit fly species showed LC_{50}s ranging between 10 200 and 13 340 mg/litre of nutrient media. The LC_{50} for third instar mosquito larvae (*Aedes aegypti*) was 25–120 mg/litre in a 4-h static test.

The effects on plants of exposure to 2-propanol at concentrations between 2100 mg/litre and more than 36 000 mg/litre ranged from no effect to complete inhibition of germination.

1.7 Effects on Experimental Animals and *In Vitro* Test Systems

The acute toxicity of 2-propanol for mammals, based on mortality, is low, whether exposure is via the oral, dermal, or respiratory route. The LD_{50} values for several animal species after oral administration varied between 4475 and 7990 mg/kg body weight; the inhalation 8-h LC_{50}s for rats ranged from 46 000 to 55 000 mg/m^3 air. At these lethal levels, rats showed severe irritation of the mucous membranes and severe depression of the central nervous system. Death was caused by respiratory or cardiac arrest. Histopathological lesions included congestion and oedema of the lungs, and cell degeneration in the liver.

Single oral doses of 3000 or 6000 mg 2-propanol/kg body weight resulted in a reversible accumulation of triglycerides in the liver of rats. Microsomal enzyme induction was observed in rats at an oral dose level of 390 mg/kg.

Undiluted 2-propanol appeared non-irritant when applied to the clipped or abraded skin of rabbits for 4 h. However, 2-propanol caused irritation when 0.1 ml of undiluted compound was applied to the rabbit eye. High vapour concentrations of 2-propanol caused irritation of the respiratory tract in mice, and the respiratory rate was decreased by 50% at concentrations of 12 300–43 525 mg/m^3 of air.

Repeated exposure studies on the effects of 2-propanol in animals are rather limited. After inhalation of 500 mg 2-propanol/m^3 for 5 days/week and 4 h/day over 4 months, irritation of the respiratory tract, haematological changes, and histopathological alterations in the liver and spleen were seen in rats. In another study group, 5 rats of each sex received drinking-water containing 2-propanol for 27 weeks. Comparison of animals receiving approximately 600 or 2300 mg/kg per day (males) and 1000 or 3900 mg/kg per day (females) with untreated controls showed growth retardation only in both exposed female groups. No further adverse effects were found.

The available evidence suggests that the effects of 2-propanol on the central nervous system (CNS) are similar to those of ethanol. The oral ED$_{50}$ for narcosis in rabbits is 2280 mg/kg, the intraperitoneal ED$_{50}$ for loss of righting reflex in mice is 165 mg/kg, and the intraperitoneal threshold for induction of ataxia in rats is 1106 mg/kg. These values are approximately two times lower than those for ethanol. Inhalation of 2-propanol at 739 mg/m^3 for 6 h/day, 5 days/week for 15 weeks did not result in any adverse effects in an open field test.

2-Propanol was evaluated in a 2-generation study on rats by the administration of 1290, 1380, or 1470 mg/kg per day in the drinking-water to both generations. The only adverse effect noted was a transient reduction in growth rate in the F_0 generation. In contrast, other research workers observed an increase in malformations in a teratology study after pregnant rats were dosed orally with 252 or 1008 mg 2-propanol/kg per day (maternal toxicity was not discussed). Both of these doses, administered in the drinking-water for 45 days, were also reported to increase the estrous cycle to 5 days (versus 4 days in controls). Increased total embryonic mortality was seen when female rats received drinking-water doses of 1800 mg/kg per day for 6 months prior to breeding; various effects on intrauterine and postnatal survival were reported at a dose as low as 0.18 mg/kg per day, but no consistent pattern was apparent. Pregnant rats were exposed to airborne 2-propanol at concentrations of 9001, 18 327, or 23 210 mg/m^3 (3659, 7450, or 9435 ppm). The two higher concentrations were toxic to the maternal animals, but 9001 mg/m^3 was not. Developmental toxicity was seen at all three concentrations.

2-Propanol gave negative results in a test at 0.18 mg per plate for point mutations in *S. typhimurium* and a test for sister chromatid exchange in Chinese hamster lung fibroblasts. It induced mitotic abnormalities in rat bone marrow cells and in onion root tip cells *in vitro*. No other mutagenicity data were available.

2-Propanol was tested in several limited carcinogenicity studies in the mouse using the dermal (3 times weekly for 1 year), inhalation (7700 mg/m^3 for 3–7 h/day, 5 days/week, over 5–8 months) and subcutaneous (20 mg undiluted, weekly for 20–40 weeks) routes of exposure. The occurrence of tumours was investigated in the three studies in the skin, lung, and at the injection site, respectively. There was no evidence of any carcinogenic effects. There are no adequate epidemiology data with which to assess the carcinogenicity of 2-propanol for human beings. The available data suggest that di-2-propyl sulfate, an intermediate in the strong and weak acid processes for the production of 2-propanol, may be causally associated with the induction of paranasal sinus cancer in human beings.

1.8 Health Effects in Human Beings

Several cases of intoxication have been reported after oral ingestion and also in febrile children who were sponged with 2-propanol preparations. In cases of poisoning, the major signs are those of alcoholic intoxication including nausea, vomiting, abdominal pain, gastritis, hypotension, and hypothermia. 2-Propanol depresses the central nervous system about twice as much as ethanol, causing unconsciousness, ending in deep coma; death may follow due to respiratory depression. Other compound-related effects are hyperglycaemia, elevated protein levels in cerebrospinal fluid, and atelectasis. Although skin absorption has been deemed insignificant, a case report on a child intoxicated after being sponged with 2-propanol suggested that dermal absorption should not be underestimated, particularly in children. No adverse effects were observed in healthy volunteers who drank syrup containing 2.6 or 6.4 mg 2-propanol/kg, daily, for 6 weeks. A group of male volunteers, when exposed to 2-propanol vapours at concentrations of 490, 980, or 1970 mg/m^3 air for 3–5 min, judged irritation to be "mild" at 980 mg/m^3 and to be "satisfactory" for their own 8-h occupational exposure.

Skin irritation in the form of erythema, 2nd and 3rd degree burns, and blisters was reported in premature infants following prolonged contact with 2-propanol. Occasionally, cases of allergic contact dermatitis have also been reported.

Few epidemiological studies were available on mortality from cancer or from other causes. In a group of 71 workers employed for over 5 years in a plant manufacturing 2-propanol by the strong acid process, 7 cancer cases were reported including 4 cases of paranasal sinus cancer. In a cohort study on 779 workers at a similar plant, the age- and sex- adjusted incidences of sinus and laryngeal cancer were 21 times higher than expected. The minimum latency period was 10 years. In another retrospective cohort study at another plant using the strong acid process, there were more than 4000 person-years at risk. The results showed that mortality rates due to all causes and due to neoplasms were not significantly higher than expected. A retrospective cohort study was undertaken in a plant manufacturing 2-propanol by the weak acid process. More than 11 000 person-years were at risk. The mortality rate due to all causes was lower than expected. No excess mortality due to all cancers was observed. However, the incidence of buccal and pharyngeal cancer was 4 times higher than expected. The cohort studies collectively suggest a cancer hazard related to the strong acid manufacturing process but, in two small case-control studies, no evidence of an association between exposure to 2-propanol and the incidence of gliomas or lymphatic leukaemia was reported.

There are reports suggesting that combined exposure to carbon tetrachloride and 2-propanol in workers results in potentiation of the toxicity of the former.

1.9 Summary of Evaluation

Exposure of human beings to 2-propanol may occur through inhalation during manufacture, processing, and both occupational and household use. Exposure to a potentially lethal level in the general population may result from accidental or intentional ingestion and children may be exposed when sponged with 2-propanol preparations (rubbing alcohol).

2-Propanol is rapidly absorbed and distributed throughout the body, partly as acetone. Exposure-effect data on human beings under conditions of acute overexposure are scarce and show great variation. The major effects are gastritis, depression of the central nervous system with hypothermia and respiratory depression, and hypotension. The acute mortality data on experimental animals indicate that the toxicity of 2-propanol is low, the oral LD_{50} values in various species ranging between 4475 and 7990 mg/kg, and the inhalation LC_{50} values for rats being around 50 000 mg/m^3. In rabbits 2-propanol did not irritate the skin, but the application of 0.1 ml undiluted 2-propanol irritated the eyes.

In man, the most likely acute effects of exposure to high levels of 2-propanol through ingestion or inhalation are alcoholic intoxication and narcosis.

No adequate animal studies are available from which an evaluation can be made of the human health risks associated with repeated exposure to 2-propanol. However, the results of two short-term studies on rats, including inhalation exposure (500 mg/m^3 for 4 h/day, 5 days per week, for 4 months) and oral exposure (600–3900 mg/kg in the drinking-water), suggest that exposure to 2-propanol at some of the very high occupational exposure levels reported should be avoided.

Inhalation exposure of pregnant rats to 2-propanol provided a lowest-observed-effect level (LOEL) of 18 327 mg/m^3 (7450 ppm) and a no-observed-effect level (NOEL) of 9001 mg/m^3 (3659 ppm) for maternal toxicity. In the same study, 9001 mg/m^3 (3659 ppm) was a LOEL for developmental toxicity, with no demonstration of a NOEL. These concentrations are higher than those likely to be encountered under conditions of human exposure.

Summary

2-Propanol was negative in genotoxicity tests but induced mitotic aberrations in the bone marrow of rats. Although these findings suggest that the substance does not have any genotoxic potential, no adequate assessment of mutagenicity can be made on the basis of the limited data.

The available data are inadequate to assess the carcinogenicity of 2-propanol in experimental animals. There are no data to assess the carcinogenicity of 2-propanol in human beings.

It is unlikely that 2-propanol will pose a serious health risk for the general population under exposure conditions likely to be normally encountered.

2-Propanol disappears rapidly (half-time < 2.5 days) from the atmosphere and removal of 2-propanol from water and soil occurs rapidly by aerobic and anaerobic biodegradation, especially after adaptation of initially seeded microorganisms. In view of the physical properties of 2-propanol, its potential for bioaccumulation is low. It does not present a risk to naturally occurring organisms at concentrations that usually occur in the environment.

2. IDENTITY, PHYSICAL AND CHEMICAL PROPERTIES, ANALYTICAL METHODS

2.1 Identity

Chemical formula: C_3H_8O

Chemical structure:

```
        H   H   H
        |   |   |
    H—  C — C — C  —H
        |   |   |
        H   OH  H
```

Common name: isopropyl alcohol

Common synonyms: dimethylcarbinol, isopropanol, 2-propanol (IUPAC and CAS name), propanol-2, propan-2-ol, sec-propyl-alcohol

Common trade names: Alcojel, Alcosolve 2, Avantin(e), Chromar, Combi-Schutz, E 501, Hartosol, Imsol A, IPS-1, Isohol, Lutosol, Perspirit, Petrohol, PRO, Propol, Spectrar, Takineocol, UN 1219

Abbreviation: IPA

CAS registry number: 67-63-0

Specifications: three commercial grades with different water contents are available in the USA: 91% and 95% by volume, and anhydrous 2-propanol (IARC, 1977); the anhydrous grade typically contains 99.5% or more of

Specifications: 2-propanol, and water (0.5% by weight) and
(*continued*) aldehydes and ketones (0.1% by weight as
acetone) as the main impurities [47].

Conversion 1 mg 2-propanol/m^3 air = 0.41 ppm at
factors: 25 °C and 101.3 kPa (760 mmHg);
1 ppm = 2.46 mg/m^3 air.

2.2 Physical and Chemical Properties

2-Propanol is a highly flammable liquid at room temperature and standard atmospheric pressure. Its odour resembles that of a mixture of ethanol and acetone, and its taste is slightly bitter. The compound is completely miscible with water, ethanol, acetone, chloroform, and benzene. 2-Propanol and water form a constant boiling mixture that contains 88% by weight (91% by volume) of 2-propanol and boils at 80–81 °C. 2-Propanol undergoes all chemical reactions typical of secondary alcohols. It reacts violently with strong oxidizing agents. In a fire, it may decompose to form toxic gases, such as carbon monoxide. Physical and chemical data on 2-propanol are given in Table 1.

Table 1. Some physical and chemical properties of 2-propanol

Physical state	liquid
Colour	colourless
Relative molecular mass	60.09
Odour perception threshold	7.990 mg/m3 [a]
Odour recognition threshold	18.4– 120 mg/m3 [a]
Boiling point (°C)	82
Water solubility	infinite
log *n*-octanol/water partition coefficient	0.14 [b]
Specific density (20 °C)	0.785
Relative vapour density	2.07
Vapour pressure (20 °C)	4.4 kPa (33 mmHg)
Flash point (°C)	12 (closed cup) 17 (open cup)[c]
Flammability limits	2– 12% by volume

[a] From: May [185], Oelert & Florian [196], and Hellman & Small [109].
[b] Experimentally derived by Veith et al. [262].
[c] From: Kirk & Othmer [137].

2.3 Analytical Methods

A summary of methods for the determination of 2-propanol in air, water, and biological media is presented in Table 2.

Kring et al. [144] evaluated the US NIOSH charcoal tube sampling method after having identified several shortcomings in the NIOSH validation procedure, including dry air dilution and small sample sizes, because of short sampling periods (15 min). The overall accuracy for the determination of 2-propanol was 30.4% at concentrations of 128 and 428 mg/m^3, 80% relative humidity, and sampling periods of 6 h.

The sensitivity of the gas chromatographic determination of alcohols with electron capture or photoionization detection can be greatly improved by prior derivatization with pentafluorophenyldimethylsilyl chloride [145].

Ramsey & Flanagan [211] reported a method for the detection and identification of 2-propanol and other volatile organic compounds in the headspace of blood, plasma, or serum, using gas chromatography with flame-ionization and electron-capture detection. The method is applicable to samples obtained from victims of poisoning, for which a high sensitivity is not required. After preincubation of the samples with a proteolytic enzyme, the method can be used for the analysis of tissues.

Gas chromatographic methods, using flame-ionization detection, are available for the determination of 2-propanol in milk and milk products [201], in fruits [45], in oilseed meals and flours [84], in solid fish protein [3,237], in drugs [115], and in drug raw materials [183]. The determination of C_1–C_4 alcohols in gasoline can be done by direct injection into a gas chromatograph with an ion-trap detector [231]. Another direct method for the determination of C_1–C_3 alcohols and water in gasoline is size-exclusion liquid chromatography and detection by a differential refractometry [292]. One gas chromatographic method, using thermal conductivity detection, is described for the determination of 2-propanol in aerosol products [142]. Methods for the identification of 2-propanol as flavour volatile are also described [115] (Table 6; section 5.2).

Table 2. Sampling, preparation, and determination of 2-propanol

Medium	Sampling method	Analytical method	Detection limit	Sample size	Comments	Reference
Air	sampling on charcoal, desorption by carbon disulfide containing 1% butanol	gas chromatography with flame ionization detection, packing by FFAP on Chromosorb W	0.01 mg/sample	0.0002–0.003 m^3	suitable for personal and area monitoring validated over the range of 165–3300 mg/m^3	[259]
Air	sampling on charcoal, desorption by a 1:1 mixture of carbon disulfide and water	gas chromatography with flame ionization detection, packing by Oronite NIW on Carbopack B	0.25 mg/m^3	0.024 m^3	suitable for area monitoring, applicable to mixtures of both polar and non-polar solvents	[152]
Air	sampling on porous polymer, based on 2,6-diphenyl-p-phenylene oxide, desorption by heating	gas chromatography with mass spectrometric detection and OV-101, SE-30, or SP-1000 capillary columns	0.0012 mg/m^3	0.002 m^3	suitable for area monitoring, designed for the analysis of ambient and indoor air	[123]
Air	cryogenic sampling on chromosorb WAW coated with trifluoropropylmethyl-silicone, desorption by heating	two-dimensional gas chromatography with photoionization and flame ionization detection, column 1: 1,2,3-tris(2-cyanoethoxy)-propane on Chromosorb WAW, column 2: OV-101 packed capillary	2×10^{-5} mg/m^3	0.002–0.003 m^3	suitable for area monitoring, identification of unknown compounds by mass spectrometry; designed for the analysis of a wide range of low-molecular mass compounds; oxygenates in ambient air	[126]

Table 2 (contd).

Medium	Sampling method	Analytical method	Detection limit	Sample size	Comments	Reference
Air	direct injection	photoionization-ion mobility spectrometry	0.025 mg/m^3		working range, 25–2500 mg/m^3	[154]
Water	direct injection	gas chromatography with flame ionization detection, packing by porous polymer Tenax GC	1 mg/litre	0.001 ml	applicable to a mixture of a wide variety of compounds	[139]
Water	direct injection	gas chromatography with steam as carrier and flame ionization detection, packing by Chromosorb PAW modified with phosphoric acid	0.04 mg/litre	0.002 ml	applicable to a mixture of aliphatic compounds	[256.]
Water	extraction by micro steam distillation with ethyl ether	gas chromatography with flame ionization detection, packing by Carbowax 20M; confirmation by mass spectrometry	0.2 mg/litre	50 ml	applicable to the analysis of soft drinks	[260]

Table 2 (contd).

Water	derivatization by 2-fluoro-1-methyl-pyridinium p-toluene-sulfonate in presence of tridodecylamine	paper electrophoresis with detection by Dragendorff's reagent	39 mg/litre	0.1 ml	applicable to the analysis of mixtures of primary and secondary alcohols, such as in alcoholic beverages	[20]
Blood	sampled blood placed in aluminium capsule, capsule heated in GC injector and pierced	gas chromatography with flame ionization detection, packing with Carbowax 20M on Chromosorb WAW-DMCS	1 mg/litre	0.0005 ml	headspace method	[150]
Serum	direct injection of deproteinized sample with n-propanol added as internal standard	gas chromatography with flame ionization detection, bonded methyl-silicone-coated capillary column	60 mg/litre	0.2 ml	applicable to a mixture of aliphatic alcohols and acetone	[236]
Blood, urine	headspace sampling, 1% dioxane in water added to samples as internal standard	gas chromatography with flame ionization detection, packing with Carbowax 20M on Carbopack B	not reported	0.2 ml	applicable to a mixture of aliphatic alcohols, acetone, and acetaldehyde	[180]

On the basis of the correlation found between alveolar and blood acetone levels in rats and human beings and 2-propanol exposure levels (section 6.3), it can be concluded that these acetone levels can be used for biological monitoring. Acetone concentrations in the saliva of human beings have also been shown to be well correlated with 2-propanol exposure levels [250]. Although 2-propanol levels in the breath and saliva are equally well correlated with environmental 2-propanol concentrations, the half-life of 2-propanol is much shorter than that of acetone (section 6.4).

3. SOURCES OF HUMAN AND ENVIRONMENTAL EXPOSURE

3.1 Natural Occurrence

2-Propanol has been identified as a metabolic product of a variety of microorganisms and as a flavour volatile in foodstuffs, primarily plant products (section 5).

3.2 Man-made Sources

3.2.1 Production levels and processes

2.1.1 Production levels

Estimated production capacities for 2-propanol in 1984 in the USA and western Europe were 1129 and nearly 1000 kilotonnes, respectively [72, 223], although current production may be lower. The major producers in western Europe are the Federal Republic of Germany, France, the Netherlands, and the United Kingdom, with estimated production capacities of 29, 13, 29, and 24% of the total western European capacity in 1981, respectively [137]. In the USA, real production gradually declined from 878 kilotonnes in 1976 to 550 kilotonnes in 1983 [223, 275]. Japan was reported to produce 58 kilotonnes in 1975 [120] and 96 kilotonnes in 1982 [199]. On the basis of data from Japan, western Europe, and the USA [120, 223], world production in 1975 can be estimated to have exceeded 1100 kilotonnes.

2.1.2 Production processes

2-Propanol can be produced from propene by 2 different processes, i.e., indirect hydration and direct catalytic hydration. The former process is believed to have been replaced by the direct hydration process in Japan, the USA, and in western Europe. 2-Propanol is also produced by the catalytic hydrogenation of acetone [120, 223]. Initially, indirect hydration involved the feeding of 88–93% sulfuric acid and propene gas into a reactor to produce a mixture of isopropyl and diisopropyl sulfates, which were hydrolysed with water to 2-propanol. Principal by-products were diisopropyl ether and isopropyl oils consisting mainly of polypropylenes of high relative molecular mass [257]. Acetone and other by-products of low molecular mass, as well as sulfur dioxide were formed and these gave rise to further condensation products. This so-called strong-acid process has been causally related with an excess risk of cancer of the paranasal sinuses [120] (section 9.2.1). It has gradually been replaced by the weak-acid process, in which propene gas is absorbed in, and reacted with, 60% sulfuric acid and the resulting sulfates hydrolysed in a single-step process. 2-Propanol is stripped and refined from the condensate, which also contains diisopropyl ether, acetone, and polymer oils of low relative molecular mass [257]. The current major process, catalytic hydration of propene with water, has three variants: gas-phase hydration using a fixed-bed supported phosphoric acid catalyst, a mixed-phase reaction using a cation-exchange resin catalyst, and a liquid phase reaction in the presence of a dissolved tungsten catalyst [137]. Catalytic hydration largely avoids the corrosion and effluent problems associated with the sulfuric acid processes.

3.2.2 Uses

2-Propanol is mainly used as a solvent, and in pharmaceutical, household, and personal products [14, 120, 137, 223]. It is a low-cost solvent with many consumer and industrial applications (Table 3) and it has been estimated that, in 1975, between 35 and 45% of the total consumption of 2-propanol in Japan, western Europe, and the USA, was used in this way [120]. Apart from its solvent properties, 2-propanol also possesses cooling, antipyretic, rubefacient, cleansing, and antiseptic properties [202].

2-Propanol is used in the production of acetone and its derivatives and in the manufacture of other chemicals, such as isopropyl acetate, isopropylamine, diisopropyl ether, isopropyl xanthate, fatty acid esters of 2-propanol, herbicidal esters, and aluminium isopropoxide [47, 137].

Other uses include the application of 2-propanol as: a denaturant in industrial solvents, a coolant in beer manufacture, a coupling agent, a dehydrating agent, a polymerization modifier in the production of polyvinyl fluoride, a foam inhibitor, a de-icing agent, a preservative, a heat-exchange medium, and in windscreen wiper concentrates [47, 137, 291]. It is also used as a flavouring agent in, for example, tea and beer [47, 242].

Table 3. Solvent applications of 2-propanol[a]

Function	Application
1. Process solvent	- extraction and purification of natural products, such as vegetable and animal oils and fats, gums, resins, waxes, colours, flavourings, alkaloids, vitamins, kelp and alginates - carrier in the manufacture of food products - purification, crystallization and precipitation of organic chemicals
2. Coating and dye solvent	- in synthetic polymers, such as phenolic varnishes and nitrocellulose lacquers - in cements, primers, paints, and inks
3. Cleaning and drying agent	- in the manufacture of electronic parts, for metals and photographic films and papers, in glass cleaners, liquid soaps and detergents, and in aerosols (see 5)
4. Solvent in topically applied preparations	- in pharmaceutical products: embrocations, massage solutions, such as rubbing alcohol (70% 2-propanol aerosols (see 5) - in cosmetics: hair tonics, perfumes, skin lotions, hair dye rinses and permanent wave lotions, skin cleaners and deodorants, nail polishes, shampoos
5. Aerosol solvent	- cleaners, waxes, polishes, paints, de-icers, shoe and sock sprays, insect repellants, hair sprays, deodorants, air-fresheners - medical and veterinary products: antiseptics, foot fungicides, first aid and medical vapour sprays, skin soothers, veterinary pink eye, wound, and dehorning sprays, house and garden type insecticides

[a] From: Anon. [14], CEC [47], Kirk & Othmer [137], Zakhari [291].

3.2.3 Waste disposal

2-Propanol may enter the atmosphere, water, and soil following waste disposal (section 4.1). At hazardous waste sites and landfills, 2-propanol was identified in the air and in leachate (section 5.1). Emissions of 2-propanol via waste gases and waste water occur in industry and diffuse airborne emissions will occur during the use of the compound in consumer products (section 4.1).

Air emissions can be controlled by incineration, gas stripping, or biological oxidation in biofiltration systems [72]. 2-Propanol can be removed from waste water by biodegradation (section 4.3.1). Activated carbon adsorption is not feasible as adsorption on this compound is poor [97]. Removal of the compound from waste water by reverse osmosis (hyperfiltration) can be successful, depending on the type of membrane used. Cellulose acetate membranes yielded 40–60% separation of 2-propanol, while cross-linked polyethyleneimine and aromatic polyamine membranes yielded 80–90% separation [76, 80].

Ozonization of 2-propanol appears to be too slow a process to be of any significance for water treatment [114].

4. ENVIRONMENTAL TRANSPORT, DISTRIBUTION, AND TRANSFORMATION

4.1 Transport and Distribution Between Media

In view of the physical properties and the use pattern of 2-propanol, it can be concluded that the main pathway of entry of this compound into the environment is through its emission into the atmosphere during production, handling, storage, transport, and use, and following waste disposal. Second in importance will be its emission to water and soil. In the USA, it was estimated that 1.5% of the production in 1976 was lost to the environment [74]. Emission registration data from the Netherlands over the years 1974–79 indicated that industrial airborne emissions amounted to 3.3% of the 1975 production volume, and emissions into water to 0.2%. From more recent data, a total industrial release into the environment of approximately 0.6% of the 1985 production capacity was estimated [72]. However, this figure is hardly significant, because of the wide use of 2-propanol in a considerable range of consumer products; disposal of wastes will also account for large emissions. For example, in the Netherlands, an emission factor for the domestic use of 2-propanol in aerosol sprays was estimated to be 430 mg per inhabitant per day [212]. This source alone would result in an annual emission into the air of 2.1% of the 1975 production volume [72]. In 1976 in the USA, 50% of the 2-propanol produced was estimated to be released into the atmosphere [74].

Intercompartmental transfer of 2-propanol can occur between water, soil or waste and air, and between soil or waste and water. Volatilization of the compound will be considerable in view of its rather high vapour pressure. Jones & McGugan [125] measured the evaporation rate of 2-propanol, undiluted or as a 1:1 (v/v) mixture with water, from a shallow pool or from pulverized domestic waste, under controlled conditions. The rate of evaporation of undiluted 2-propanol from a pool was 1.1 kg/m^2 per h at a wind speed of 0.5 m/second, an ambient air temperature of 12 °C, and a pool temperature of 13 °C. The evaporation rate of diluted

2-propanol was 1.5 kg/m^2 per hour at a wind speed of 4.5 m/second, a pool temperature of 20 °C, and an ambient air temperature of 22 °C. Addition of domestic waste to both the diluted and the undiluted 2-propanol initially increased the evaporation rate, but strongly attenuated the release of vapour within 2 h.

Transport of 2-propanol from the atmosphere to soil or water will occur via rain-out, as it is highly soluble in water. Data on the behaviour of 2-propanol in soil are scarce. With respect to adsorption, there is one study showing that the compound is poorly adsorbed on activated carbon [97]. Since 2-propanol is completely miscible with water, it can be expected to be very mobile in the soil [72] and it has been shown to increase the permeability of soil to aromatic hydrocarbons [81].

4.2 Abiotic Degradation

Once in the atmosphere, 2-propanol will be degraded mainly by hydroxyl radicals. It is not expected to react at appreciable rates with other reactive species, such as ozone, and hydroperoxy-, alkyl-, and alkoxy-radicals. Since the compound does not absorb ultraviolet radiation within the solar spectrum, photolysis is not expected [46]. Experimentally determined rate constants for the reaction between 2-propanol and hydroxyl radicals are 0.71×10^{-11} ml/molecule per second at 32 °C [164], and 0.54×10^{-11} ml/molecule per second at 23 °C [200]. On the basis of these rate constants, atmospheric residence times of 1.4 and 2.3 days, respectively, can be calculated [61]. These short lifetimes will prevent migration of the chemical into the stratosphere.

The initial reaction product of 2-propanol with a hydroxy radical is an α-hydroxy-2-propyl radical. By analogy with the irradiation of 2-butanol in an NO_x--air atmosphere, these radicals are expected to react with oxygen almost exclusively with hydrogen abstraction from the hydroxyl-group to produce acetone, or with loss of methyl to give acetaldehyde. Follow-up reactions will produce small quantities of peroxyacetyl nitrate, formaldehyde, methyl nitrate, and formic acid [46].

Hydrolysis or light-induced degradation of 2-propanol in water cannot be expected. No data are available on abiotic degradation in soil.

4.3 Biotransformation

4.3.1 Biodegradation

The results of the determination of the biological oxygen demand (BOD) by dilution methods at 20 °C are summarized in Table 4. Unless otherwise stated, the results are expressed as a percentage of the theoretical oxygen demand (ThOD), which is 2.40 g oxygen/g 2-propanol. The chemical oxygen demand (COD) was reported to be 96 and 93% of the ThOD by Price et al. [208] and Bridie et al. [33], respectively.

Table 4. BOD and COD of 2-propanol

Dilution water	Source or seed	Adaptation (+/-)	BOD_x[a]	Value (% of ThOD)	Reference
Fresh	municipal waste water	-	BOD_5	7	[289]
		-	BOD_{20}	70	
	domestic waste water	-	BOD_5	28	[208]
		-	BOD_{20}	78	
	domestic waste water	-	BOD_5	66	[268]
	domestic waste water	-	BOD_5	74	[269]
	activated sludge	+	BOD_5	99[b]	[203]
	effluent from a biological waste treatment plant	+	BOD_5	72	[33]
		-	BOD_5	49	
Salt	domestic waste water	-	BOD_5	13	[208]
		-	BOD_{20}	72	

[a] BOD_x = biological oxygen demand after x days of incubation.
[b] Expressed as percentage of the COD.

Adaptation of the seed material to the chemical enhances the rate of biodegradation considerably. Gerhold & Malaney [95] added 2-propanol to undiluted activated sludge and found an oxygen uptake of 10% of the ThOD in 24 h. Mack [175] measured total degradation of 2-propanol within 96 h and total degradation of the initial product acetone within 120–144 h following incubation in a standard medium that had been inoculated by effluent from a water purification plant. In another study, 2-propanol (50 mg/litre) was added as the sole source of carbon to a mineral medium in a continuous flow reactor, seeded by a culture isolated from activated sludge using methanol, phenol, acetone, and 2-propanol as substrates. Growth was extremely poor. However, when acetone (100 mg/litre) was added as well, almost 100% degradation of the 2 chemicals was achieved within a minimum of 2.9 h. The authors concluded that, in this case, the oxidation of 2-propanol was dependent on the simultaneous oxidation of acetone. When 2-propanol was added to the same medium, seeded by a culture isolated using 2-propanol as the sole substrate, almost 100% degradation was achieved within a minimum of 4.3 h [281].

In a water treatment facility of a plant manufacturing organic chemicals, a typical removal efficiency for 2-propanol was 76%, using an aerated, non-flocculent, biological stabilization process [25]. After conversion to an activated sludge facility, the removal efficiency increased to 96% [147].

There are two reports on anaerobic biodegradation. Typical 2-propanol removal efficiencies for an anaerobic lagoon treatment facility, with a retention time of 15 days, were 50% after loading with dilute waste, and 69 and 74% after loading with concentrated wastes [118]. In closed bottle studies, 2-propanol was completely degraded anaerobically by an acetate-enriched culture, derived from a seed of domestic sludge. The culture started to use cross-fed 2-propanol, after 4 days, at a rate of 200 mg/litre per day. In a mixed reactor with a 20-day retention time, seeded by the same culture, 56% removal was achieved in the 20 days following 70 days of acclimation to a final 2-propanol concentration of 10 000 mg/litre [55].

4.3.2 Bioaccumulation

2-Propanol is completely miscible with water. Its log n-octanol/water partition coefficient is 0.14 [263]. A bioconcentration factor of 0.5 can be calculated using the formula of Veith & Kosian [262]. In addition, the compound is biodegradable. In view of these data, no bioaccumulation is expected.

5. ENVIRONMENTAL LEVELS AND HUMAN EXPOSURE

5.1 Environmental Levels

The rapid removal of 2-propanol from air and water is reflected in the few reports indicating its presence in these compartments (sections 4.2 and 4.3). No data are available on the occurrence of the compound in soil.

2-Propanol was detected, at a level of 95 mg/m^3 air, at the outlet of the main chimney of a paint-manufacturing plant in France in 1980. The compound was not detected at a distance of 10–30 m from this chimney [51]. In 1970, Gorlova [98] reported that average atmospheric levels of 2-propanol at distances of 500 and 5000 m from a plant producing 2-propanol by indirect hydration, were 1.7 and 0.2 mg/m^3 air, with maxima of 3 and 0.5 mg/m^3 air, respectively. In 260 1-h samples of air from 4 sites in Stockholm, Sweden, in 1983, 2-propanol concentrations ranging between 0.61 and 108 mg/m^3 were measured with averages of between 1.52 and 35.2 mg/m^3. In 56 air samples from a monitoring site near dense traffic 12 km outside central Stockholm, concentrations of between 0.12 and 2.93 mg/m^3 were measured, the average being 0.74 mg/m^3. The 2-propanol levels were not correlated with typical vehicle exhaust compound levels. However, a correlation was found between 2-propanol levels and the use of anti-freezing agents for windscreen washers at a similar site [126].

2-Propanol was detected in the air beneath the surface of 2 out of 6 landfill sites sampled in the United Kingdom. At these 2 sites, used for the disposal of domestic waste, the 2-propanol concentrations were 17 mg/m^3 and more than 46 mg/m^3, respectively [288]. Analysis of a total of 82 air samples at 5 hazardous waste sites in New Jersey, USA, revealed the presence of 2-propanol at 4 sites [151]. Leaching from landfills may result in ground water pollution. In 1982–83, 2-propanol concentrations of up to 8.8 mg/litre water were measured in 6 out of 7 samples of leachate, obtained from test wells in 1 of 5 landfills sampled in the United Kingdom [225].

2-Propanol has been identified as a metabolic product in microorganisms, as shown in Table 5.

Table 5. 2-Propanol production by microorganisms

Type	Species	Reference
Aerobic fish spoilage bacteria	*Pseudomonas* spp., *Moraxella*-like, *Flavobacterium, Micrococcus,* Coryneforms, *Vibrio*	[7]
Aerobic beef spoilage bacteria	*Pseudomonas* spp.	[63]
Aerobic potato tuber soft rot bacteria	*Erwinia carotovora*	[273]
Anaerobic bacteria	*Clostridium beijerinckii* *Clostridium aurantibutyricum*	[92]
Anaerobic methylotrophic, propane fed bacteria		[181]
Fungi, mushroom	*Leucocoprinus elaedis*	[93]
Yeast	*Kluyveromyces lactis*	[107]

5.2 General Population Exposure

5.2.1 Exposure via food

When 2-propanol is used as an extraction or carrier solvent for food constituents, the compound may be found in the final product. It was detected in 8 out of 17 samples of lemonade, prepared with natural essence extracted with 2-propanol. Concentrations of between 0.2 and 82 mg/litre were measured in 7 samples and 325 mg/litre in one sample [260]. The compound was also identified in fish protein concentrate, extracted by 2-propanol [237]. The Scientific Committee for Food of the Commission of the European Communities has published industry-derived residue levels in foodstuffs following the use of 2-propanol as an extraction and/or carrier solvent. Typical levels are: 250 mg/kg of dry fish protein concentrate, 50 mg/kg of meat product as consumed, 750 mg/kg of meat after use of 2-propanol as a smoke flavour carrier and before drying, 1200 mg/kg of jam, and 3000 mg/kg of jelly [47].

Studies showing the presence of 2-propanol as a flavour volatile in a variety of foodstuffs are summarized in Table 6.

Microbial metabolism may be responsible for the presence of 2-propanol in certain foodstuffs, such as cheese, as suggested by Bosset & Liardon [31]. Approximately 25% of the 2-propanol found in beer is added as a flavouring agent during its manufacture [242].

5.2.2 Exposure via other consumer products

The general population is potentially exposed to a wide variety of consumer products containing 2-propanol (section 3.2.2). In a 1980 survey in Japan, commercial heterogeneous solvent products were collected throughout the country. Of 102 products, 12 out of 59 samples of paint, 6 out of 18 samples of ink, 1 out of 12 samples of adhesives, and 3 out of 13 samples of other products contained 2-propanol [146]. Not surprisingly, 2-propanol was one of over 250 compounds found in the indoor air of homes in 2 urban areas of the USA, where the levels were all less than 0.25 mg/m^3 [123].

Intentional or accidental poisoning by 2-propanol in consumer products has been reported frequently. Several cases will be discussed in section 9.1. The subject of non-beverage alcohol use has been reviewed recently by Egbert et al. [77], who reported that 10–15% of a specified group of alcoholics in the USA (admitted to a Veteran Administration detoxication unit) were found to have consumed non-beverage alcohols. Addiction to a disinfectant containing 2-propanol was reported in one case [133]. In Canada, the incidence of cases of exposure to 2-propanol in rubbing alcohol reported to the Poison Control Centres increased from 254 in 1973 to 338 in 1976 [151]. Rubbing alcohol is also the single most frequent source of 2-propanol intoxication in small children. This can occur from accidental ingestion, or via inhalation following sponging for fever reduction [163].

Table 6. 2-Propanol as a flavour volatile in foodstuffs

Foodstuff		Reference
Common name	Scientific name	
Reunion geranium oil	*Pelargonium roseum* Bourbon	[249]
Rooibos tea	*Asphalathus linearis*	[104]
Winged bean (raw/roasted) Soybean (raw/roasted)	*Psophocarpus tetragonolobus* *Glycine max*	[70]
Virginia peanut (raw)		[166]
Peanut (raw/roasted)	*Arachis hypogaea*	[156]
Filbert (roasted)	*Corylus avellana*	[136]
Babaco fruit	*Carica pentagona*	[229]
Apple Tomato	*Malus* *Lycopersicum*	[242]
Endive	*Cichorium endivia*	[99]
Lime essence	*Citrus arantifolia*	[189]
Grapefruit essence Grapefruit aroma oil	*Citrus paradisi*	[58]
Mushroom (fresh/edible)	*Leucocoprinus elaedis*	[93]
Kefir culture Yoghurt culture		[201]
Swiss Gruyere cheese		[31]
Feta cheese		[116]

5.3 Occupational Exposure

Workers are potentially exposed to 2-propanol during production of the compound itself or of acetone and other derivatives, or during its use in solvent type applications. In the USA, NIOSH estimated, on the basis of the 1980–83 National Occupational Exposure Survey, that over 1.8 million workers, of whom over 1.1 million were females, were potentially exposed to this compound [259]. Inhalation exposure of workers in various industries where 2-propanol or 2-propanol-containing products are used, is summarized in Table 7. In most cases, these workers were also exposed to other chemicals. No data are available on the exposure of workers in 2-propanol- or acetone-producing industries, except for the report of Guseinov [103] pertaining to a plant in the USSR producing 2-propanol by indirect hydration.

Table 7. Occupational inhalation exposure to 2-propanol

Job description (number of workers)	Country	Sampling	Concentration (mg/m^3)	Reference
Car painting (40)	Finland	personal	7.1 (average) 209 (maximum)	[148]
Printing (12)	Italy	area	8–647 15–493 (time-weighted average)	[41]
Ink production (41)	Italy	area	6.3–32.8	[42]
Paint manufacture (3)	Sweden	personal	6–258 (time-weighted average) 129 (time-weighted average – average)	[168]
Work in hospital operating theatre	United Kingdom	area	8.8 (average) 30 (maximum)	[106]
Tractor painting (28)	USA	personal area	ND^a–697 33–332	[102]
Higher aromatic booth spray painting (14)	USA	personal	4.7 (time-weighted average – average) 32 (time-weighted average – maximum) 54 (maximum)	[279]
Lower aromatic booth spray painting (16)	USA	personal	10.6 (time-weighted average – average) 125 (time-weighted average – maximum) 605 (maximum)	[279]

Table 7 (contd).

Job description (number of workers)	Country	Sampling	Concentration (mg/m^3)	Reference
Solvent wiping (11)	USA	personal	2.5 (time-weighted average – average) 13 (maximum)	[279]
Paint mixing (3)	USA	personal	4.2 (time-weighted average – average) 10 (maximum)	[276]
Spraying paint, lacquer,	USA	personal	<2.5 (time-weighted average – average)	[177]
Printing (26)	USA	personal	396 (time-weighted average – average)	[177]
Printing (2)	USA	personal	33–67	[140]
Printing (7)	USA	personal area	85–293 236	[101]
Printing (4)	USA	personal area	0.5–3.7 2.2–16.5	[152]
Printing (8)	USA	personal area	ND^a–519 15–307	[282]
Printed circuit boards manufacture (5)	USA	personal	5.8–23	[280]
Furniture stripping (7)	USA	personal	42–160	[179]

Table 7. (contd).

Degreasing metal (14)	USA	personal	2.2–10.6	[271]
Manufacture of rubber weather strips (67)	USA	personal area	ND^a–34 6.5–140	[278]
Chemicals packaging	USA	area	150–1350	[83]
2-Propanol production	USSR	area area	92 (average)^b 165 (average)^c	[103]
Chloramphenicol production	USSR	area	10–36 (average)^d ND^a–120	[173]
Sulfite additive production	USSR	area	7.1–14.6 (average)	[17]

^{a} ND = not detected.
^{b} Wintertime.
^{c} Summertime.
^{d} Average of the positive samples.

6. KINETICS AND METABOLISM

6.1 Absorption

6.1.1 Animals

Exposure of dogs, rabbits, and rats via various routes resulted in detectable levels of 2-propanol in the blood within 0.5 h of the start of the exposure [1, 121, 150, 151,158, 181, 195].

Maximum blood concentrations of 2-propanol of up to 2950 µg/litre were attained in dogs within 0.5–2 h following single oral doses of the compound in water of up to 2940 mg/kg body weight. The blood concentration was directly related to the dose level [158]. Following single oral dosing of rats with 2-propanol in water at 2000 mg/kg body weight [121] or 6000 mg/kg body weight [195], peak blood concentrations were 1080 µg/litre after 1 h and 4800–6000 µg/litre after 8 h, respectively. Apparently, gastrointestinal absorption is delayed at high doses.

Blood levels of 2-propanol were determined in groups of 3 adult (200–300 g) female Sprague-Dawley rats following 1, 10, or 19 consecutive 7-h daily exposures to measured concentrations of 7636, 18 327, or 23 210 mg/m^3 (3104, 7450, or 9435 ppm). Immature (approximately 90 g) females of the same strain were also evaluated following a single 7-h exposure to 23 210 mg/m^3 (9435 ppm). In the immature females, the blood level of 2-propanol averaged 9600 µg/litre. The blood levels in adult rats following a single exposure were not detectable at 7636 mg/m^3 (3104 ppm), 6800 µg/litre at 18 327 mg/m^3 (7450 ppm), and 7900 µg/litre at 23 210 mg/m^3 (9435 ppm). Following 10 and 19 consecutive daily exposures, blood levels in adult rats were consistently not detected at 7636 mg/m^3 (3104 ppm); 5800 and 5700 µg/litre at 18 327 mg/m^3 (7450 ppm), and 7000 and 6400 µg/litre at 23 210 (9435 ppm) [193], respectively. The Task Group noted that these blood 2-propanol levels appeared to be exceptionally high.

When rats inhaled 2-propanol at concentrations of between 1230 and 19 680 mg/m^3 for 4 or 8 h, maximum blood concentrations attained at the end of the exposure period at the highest exposure level were 235 and 760 μg/litre, respectively [151].

Wax et al. [274] injected equal volumes of 2-propanol in saline into each of several ligated loops of the intestines and into the stomach loop of anaesthetized dogs. The concentration of the solutions varied, the total dose always being 980 mg/kg body weight. Absorption from the intestines was 67–91% of the dose within 30 min and 99% within 2 h. Absorption from the stomach loop was 41% within 30 min.

Rats exposed intraperitoneally to 1000 mg 2-propanol/kg body weight in saline showed peak blood concentrations of 1020–1300 μg/litre within 1 h [1, 195].

Groups of 3 rabbits received 2-propanol in water orally at 2 or 4 mg/kg body weight or were exposed to 2-propanol in towels, one applied to the chest and others on the floor of the inhalation chamber, with or without a plastic layer to prevent skin contact. The highest blood levels of 2-propanol were produced by the oral exposures, followed by the combined dermal and inhalation exposure [181].

6.1.2 Human beings

Ten human volunteers drank orange juice containing doses of 3.75 mg 2-propanol/kg and 1200 mg ethanol/kg body weight over a period of 2 h. At the end of this period, the average peak blood concentration of 2-propanol was 0.83 ± 0.34 (mean ± standard deviation) mg/litre. When the blood was analysed after incubation with aryl sulfatase (EC 3.1.6.1), an average peak concentration of 2.27 ± 1.43 mg/litre was measured 1 h after exposure [27]. These data provide limited evidence for the sulfation of 2-propanol.

Brugnone et al. [41] analysed the alveolar air, blood, and urine of 12 printing workers, exposed to 2-propanol at concentrations of between 8 and 647 mg/m^3 air. The alveolar 2-propanol concentration was highly correlated with the exposure level at any time of exposure, the ratio of the two concentrations being 0.418. The alveolar uptake (0.03–6.6 mg/min) showed a linear increase with exposure levels.

6.2 Distribution

6.2.1 Animals

2-Propanol, a compound with infinite water solubility, is rapidly distributed throughout the body [1].

Wax et al. [274] recovered 2-propanol from the blood, spinal fluid, liver, kidneys, and brain of dogs, 30 min after exposure via injection into ligated loops of the gastrointestinal tract. Three hours after a single oral exposure of rats, the compound was found in the blood, liver, kidneys, and brain [121]. No other tissues were analysed in either study.

The permeability of the blood–brain barrier for 2-propanol was investigated in monkeys and rabbits. Anaesthetized monkeys received a single injection of 0.2 ml of an ^{11}C-labelled alcohol in the carotid artery, followed by an injection of ^{15}O-labelled water. At a cerebral blood flow of 50 ml/100 g per min, about 99% of 2-propanol, 97% of ethanol, and 93% of labelled water exchanged freely with the brain during a single capillary transit. On the basis of these data, the blood–brain barrier permeabilities for these three compounds were estimated to be 5, 2.5, and 1.8×10^{-4} cm/second, respectively [209].

6.2.2 Human beings

Following ingestion of an unknown amount of rubbing alcohol, 2-propanol as well as its metabolite acetone were found in the spinal fluid of 2 persons at levels similar to those in the serum [5, 191].

6.3 Metabolism

6.3.1 Animals

The metabolism and elimination of 2-propanol in mammals is summarized in Fig. 1. It has been well established that 2-propanol is metabolized to acetone in the rat, dog, and rabbit [1, 121, 150, 151, 195, 224, 232]. Oral (0.2, 1.0 ml) and inhalation exposure (1230–19 680 mg/m^3, for 4 h)(500–8000 ppm) of rats produced dose-related increases in blood levels of 2-propanol and its metabolite acetone. Following inhalation, the acetone/2-propanol ratio in blood decreased with increasing 2-propanol concentrations indicating saturation of the oxidative metabolic pathway above concentrations of approximately 9840 mg/m^3 (4000 ppm) [150, 151].

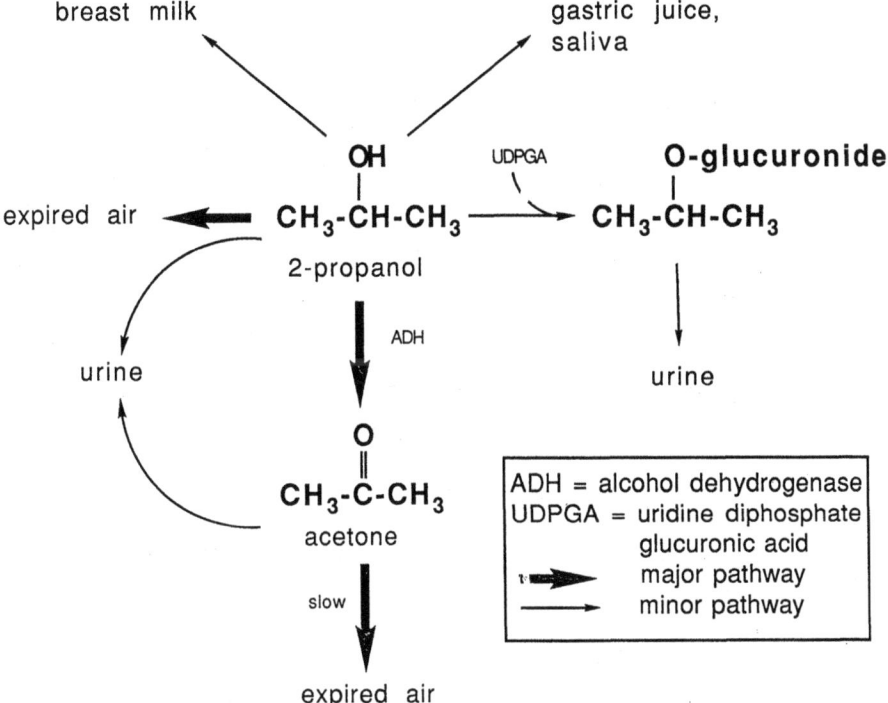

Fig. 1. Metabolism and elimination of 2-propanol in mammals.

Since adequate balance studies have not been conducted, the extent of this metabolism to acetone is not known. Siebert et al. [232] injected 750 or 1300 mg/kg body weight intravenously in rabbits and estimated that 64–84% of the dose was oxidized to acetone, confirming the earlier findings of Pohl [204].

Evidence of another metabolic pathway was found in rabbits given an oral dose of 2-propanol of 3000 mg/kg body weight, 10.2% of the dose was found in the urine as β-isopropyl-glucuronide [129].

Sufficient evidence is available to show that 2-propanol is oxidized to acetone mainly by the non-specific cytosolic enzyme alcohol dehydrogenase (ADH) (EC 1.1.1.1). When either pyrazole or 4-methylpyrazole (inhibitors of ADH) was administered to rats prior to exposure to 2-propanol, both the elimination of 2-propanol and the production of acetone were retarded [121, 193]. The elimination of 2-propanol by rats was retarded when it was given in combination with ethanol; both compounds are substrates for ADH [2, 121]. Enzyme kinetic data show that 2-propanol is a poorer substrate of ADH than ethanol. *In vitro*, the Michaelis-Menten constant (K_m) for horse liver ADH was 0.0126 mol/litre, using 2-propanol as a substrate, and 0.00018 mol/litre, using ethanol as a substrate [64]. For rat liver ADH *in vivo*, K_m was 0.034 mol/litre, using 2-propanol as a substrate, and 0.00192 mol/litre, using ethanol as a substrate. The maximum initial velocity (V_{max}) of rat liver ADH and the substrate 2-propanol *in vivo* was 1.7 times less than that with the substrate ethanol. It was further shown that the ratio of the relative rates of oxidation of 2-propanol and deuterated 2-propanol-d_7 were about the same *in vitro* and *in vivo*. From this, it can be concluded that ADH activity is the rate-limiting factor in 2-propanol metabolism [54].

It has been shown that rat liver microsomal oxidases are also capable of oxidizing 2-propanol, but that the compound is not an effective substrate for the peroxidative activity of catalase (EC 1.11.1.6) [48, 193].

6.3.2 Human beings

Acetone has also been found in the blood of human beings after exposure to 2-propanol [e.g., 11, 41, 65, 131]. Furthermore, acetone was detected in the spinal fluid, at levels similar to those in serum, in 2 persons after ingestion of 2-propanol [5, 191].

In the investigations of Brugnone et al. [41] (section 6.1.2), elevated acetone levels were measured in the blood, alveolar air, and urine of 12 printing workers. 2-Propanol was not detected in the blood or urine. The concentrations of acetone ranged between 0.76 and 15.6 mg/litre in the blood and between 3 and 93 mg/m^3 in the alveolar air. The acetone levels in alveolar air and blood increased with the increasing exposure period and were linearly related to the alveolar 2-propanol levels. Urinary acetone levels ranged from 0.85 to 53.7 mg/litre in overnight pooled urine samples and were highly correlated with the alveolar 2-propanol uptake and with blood acetone levels. Pulmonary and renal clearance of acetone were 41–97 and 0.1–3 ml/min, respectively, for 8 of the workers, showing that acetone is mainly excreted via the lungs. Pulmonary acetone excretion varied from 10.7 to 39.8% of the uptake and was inversely related to the exposure level [41]. It is known that the metabolic capacity of the human liver for acetone is limited [161].

2-Propanol and acetone have also been found in the returns of gastric lavage [5] and in saliva [250]. Reabsorption may follow excretion via these routes.

When 10 volunteers drank orange juice containing doses that gave 3.75 mg 2-propanol and 1200 mg ethanol/kg body weight over 2 h, 2-propanol was detected in the blood, partly as sulfate (section 6.1.2), and in the urine, partly as glucuronide. The total urinary excretion of 2-propanol was 1.9% of the dose [27, 28].

Human data support the importance of the ADH pathway for the oxidation of 2-propanol as observed in experimental animals. In the studies of Bonte et al. [27, 28] described above, 2-propanol was only detected in the blood when ethanol was ingested simultaneously, indicating a retarded elimination. Among 74 persons intoxicated by 2-propanol, significantly lower acetone values were found in the blood of those who had also been exposed to ethanol [11, 131]. In *in vitro* studies, the activity of human ADH with 2-propanol was 9–10% of the activity of the enzyme with ethanol as substrate [121].

Endogenous formation of 2-propanol has been revealed at autopsies of individuals not previously exposed to this compound. This observation and the results of additional studies on rats show that 2-propanol can result from the reduction of acetone by liver ADH, especially when high levels of acetone and high $NADH/NAD^+$ ratios occur. Such conditions are found in diabetes mellitus, starvation, high fat feeding, chronic alcoholism, and dehydration [68, 161, 248].

6.4 Elimination and Excretion

6.4.1 Animals

In a review article, Rietbrock & Abshagen [218] concluded that urinary excretion of both 2-propanol and its metabolite acetone is limited and in each case does not exceed 4% of the dose in the rat, rabbit, and dog. The major route of excretion is via the lungs. 2-Propanol is excreted via the gastric juice and saliva in the dog [158] and through breast milk in the rat, as shown by tissue levels in the newborn [159].

The disappearance of 2-propanol from the blood of experimental animals was found to be a first-order process at doses < 1500 mg/kg [1, 232]. In rats, the half-life of 2-propanol was 1.5 h at an intraperitoneal dose of 500 mg/kg body weight and increased to 2.5 h at a dose of 1500 mg/kg body weight. This can be explained by a limited metabolic capacity as suggested in section 6.3.1 [218]. Simultaneous administration of ethanol to rats increased the half-life of 2-propanol in the blood approximately 5-fold following acute exposure [2]. A half-life of 4 h was determined in dogs administered 1000 mg 2-propanol/kg body weight intravenously [1].

The biotransformation of 2-propanol and the elimination of the acetone produced are both slow processes. Peak acetone levels in the blood of various species, following single exposures via different routes, were only reached several hours after exposure, though acetone was already detectable shortly after the start of exposure [1, 121, 150, 151, 193, 232]. The elimination of acetone in the dog and the rat was found to be a first-order process with half-lives of 11 and 5 h, respectively [1].

After prolonged administration of 2-propanol to dogs [159] and rats [224], the elimination rate of 2-propanol was increased. Simultaneous exposure of rats to ethanol in the drinking-water (5%) and atmospheric 2-propanol at 738 mg/m^3 (300 ppm) for 5–21 weeks significantly increased the rates of elimination of 2-propanol and acetone [224].

6.4.2 Human beings

The elimination of 2-propanol in human beings also appears to follow first-order kinetics. In two alcoholics who had ingested rubbing alcohol, 2-propanol was eliminated from the blood with half-lives of 2.5 and 3 h, respectively. Acetone levels declined slowly over the next 30 h; no ethanol was detected [65]. A half-life of 2-propanol of 6.4 h was determined in a non-alcoholic, who also had ingested rubbing alcohol. The acetone level in the blood reached a maximum 30 h after admission to hospital. The half-life of acetone was 22 h. Ethanol was also found in the blood. The differences in the half-lives in these three cases may reflect metabolic adaptation in the alcoholics, or genetic variations in ADH [191].

When 4 volunteers ingested an artificial liquor containing 40% 2-propanol, acetone was detectable in exhaled air from 15 min after exposure and in the urine from 1 h after exposure [132].

7. EFFECTS ON ORGANISMS IN THE ENVIRONMENT

7.1 Aquatic Organisms

A summary of acute aquatic toxicity data is presented in Table 8. The concentration of 2-propanol was reported to have been measured in only 3 of the studies [34, 111, 263] and in no case were potential metabolites considered. In view of the volatility of the compound, it can be expected that the toxic effects observed in the other open systems studied occurred at lower concentrations than the nominal ones.

Several short- and long-term studies have also been conducted. Seiler et al. [227] determined the breakpoint of bioinhibition for a total of 20 strains of bacterial groups prevalent in a waste-water treatment plant in the chemical industry, i.e., *Zoogloea, Alcaligenes,* and *Pseudomonas*. After one week of static exposure to 2-propanol in an open system at 30 °C, 100% growth inhibition occurred at concentrations of 80 000–100 000 mg/litre of medium. No analysis for the compound was reported. The cell multiplication of blue algae (*Microcystis aeruginosa*) and green algae (*Scenedesmus quadricauda*) was just inhibited after 8 days of static exposure to 1000 and 1800 mg/litre water, respectively, in a closed system at 27 °C and a pH of 7 [35, 37]. When water fleas (*Daphnia magna*) were exposed to 2-propanol for 16 days in a semi-static test at 19 °C and a water hardness of 100 mg $CaCO_3$/litre, the highest concentration that did not result in a significant reduction in growth was 141 mg/litre water. The water was analysed for the compound just before and after each renewal of test solution [111]. A 7-day LC_{50} of 7060 mg 2-propanol/litre water was determined for 2–3-month-old guppies (*Poecilia reticulata*) in a semi-static test. No analysis for 2-propanol was reported for this open system [141].

Table 8. Acute aquatic toxicity of 2-propanol

Organism	Description	Temperature (°C)	pH	Dissolved oxygen (mg/litre)	Hardness (mg CaCO$_3$/litre)	Stat/flow open/closed[a]	Exposure period	Parameter	Nominal concentration (mg/litre)	Reference
FRESHWATER										
Bacteria	*Pseudomonas putida*	25	7			stat, closed	16 h	TT[b]	1 050	[37]
Microorganisms	activated sludge	21	7.4–8			stat, closed	3 h	50% inhibition of respiration rate	1 000	[138]
Protozoa	*Entosiphon sulcatum*	25	6.9			stat, closed	72 h	TT[b]	4 930	[36]
Protozoa	*Chilomonas paramecium*	20	6.9			stat, closed	48 h	TT[b]	104	[40]
Protozoa	*Uronema parduczi*	25	6.9			stat, closed	20 h	TT[b]	3 425	[38]
Crustacea	water flea (*Daphnia magna*)	20	8	2	250	stat, open	24 h	EC$_{50}$[c] EC$_0$ EC$_{100}$	9 714 5 102 10 000	[39]

53

Table 8 (contd).

Organism	Description	Temperature (°C)	pH	Dissolved oxygen (mg/litre)	Hardness (mg CaCO$_3$/litre)	Stat/flow open/closed[a]	Exposure period	Parameter	Nominal concentration (mg/litre)	Reference
Crustacea	water flea (*Daphnia magna*)	22			100	stat	44 h	EC$_{50}$[c,d]	2 285	[110]
Amphibia	frog tadpole (*Rana pipiens*)	20				stat		threshold narcotic concentration	22 530	[190]
Fish	fathead minnow (*Pimephales promelas*)	18–22		4		stat, open	96 h 24 h	LC$_{50}$ LC$_{50}$	11 130 11 160	[184]
Fish	fathead minnow (*Pimephales promelas*)	25	7.5	5	45	flow, open	96 h	LC$_{50}$	9 640–10 400[f]	[262]
Fish	goldfish (*Carassius auratus*)	20	6–8	4	280	stat, open	24 h	LC$_{50}$	5 000[f]	[34]

Table 8 (contd).

Fish	golden orfe (*Leuciscus idus melanotus*)	20	7-8	5	200–300	stat	48 h	LC_{50}	8 970	[127]
Fish	harlequin fish (*Rasbora heteromorpha duncker*)	20	8.1		20	flow, open	96 h	LC_{50}	4 200	[251]
							96 h	LC_{10}	1 500	
Fish	Creek chub (*Semotilus atromaculatus*)	15–21	8.3		98	stat, open	24 h	LC_0	900	[96]
SEA WATER										
Bacteria	*Photobacterium phosphoreum*	15	7			stat, closed	2 min	TT^h	15 000	[43]
		15				stat, closed	5 min	50% light reduction	35 000 42 000	[44, 62]
Worm	*Tubifex tubifex*	20				stat	2 min	EC-100^c	51 080	[56]

Table 8 (contd).

Organism	Description	Temperature (°C)	pH	Dissolved oxygen (mg/litre)	Hardness (mg CaCO₃/litre)	Stat/flow open/closed[a]	Exposure period	Parameter	Nominal concentration (mg/litre)	Reference
Crustacea	Brine shrimp (*Artemia salina*)	24				stat, open	24 h	LC_{50}	10 000	[208]
Crustacea	Brown shrimp (*Crangon crangon*)					semi-stat, open	96 h	LC_{50}	1 150	[26]

[a] Static or flow-through test; open or closed system.
[b] TT = toxic threshold for inhibition of cell multiplication.
[c] Effect is complete immobilization.
[d] Calculated value based on a quantitative structure-activity relationship between the *n*-octanol/water partition coefficient of a group of 19 organic chemicals and their anaesthetic potency.
[e] Concentration at which touching the tadpoles failed to cause motion; exposure period and conditions; and the method of calculation of the threshold not specified.
[f] Analysis for 2-propanol reported.
[g] Test compound was Imsol A (90% 2-propanol, remainder unknown).
[h] TT = toxic threshold for light reduction.

7.2 Terrestrial Organisms

7.2.1 Microorganisms

The sensitivity of 4 soil fungi, i.e., *Chrysosporium crassitunicatum*, *Nannizzia fulva*(+), *Nannizzia fulva*(−), and *Trichophyton equinum*, to saturated 2-propanol vapour was determined at 28 °C and a pH of 7. Mycelial growth of *Chrysosporium* was stimulated after 14 days of exposure, while that of the other strains was inhibited. Sporulation was poor in *Chrysosporium* and in *Trichophyton*, and fair or good in the other strains [233].

7.2.2 Insects

The 4-h LC_{50} for third instar mosquito larvae (*Aedes aegypti*) was 25 120 mg/litre water in a static test at 22–24 °C [143]. The 48-h LC_{50} values for the fruit fly strains *Drosophila melanogaster* and *Drosophila simulans* were between 10 200 and 13 340 mg/litre of nutrient medium in static tests [66]. Exposure of *Drosophila melanogaster* eggs and larvae to 7850 mg 2-propanol/litre of nutrient medium caused an 87% decrease in the activity of the non-specific enzyme alcohol dehydrogenase (EC 1.1.1.1) in the 14-day-old larvae. At the same time, viability was decreased by 74%. The development of *Drosophila simulans* was completely inhibited at the same concentration. Gas chromatographic analysis revealed that, after 4 days of exposure, acetone appeared as the 2-propanol concentration decreased. The appearance of acetone was associated with an observed decrease in enzyme activity [265]. Anderson & McDonald [13] also found a decrease in the specific activity of alcohol dehydrogenase in *Drosophila melanogaster* after 1–4 days of exposure to 2-propanol. On the other hand, they found that the stability and concentration of the enzyme increased. The authors explained the findings as an adaptation of the fruit fly to its environment.

7.2.3 Plants

The effects of 2-propanol on the rate of seed germination were investigated on several occasions. Total inhibition of the germination of barley grains was reached after incubation for 4 days at

18 °C on filter papers, absorbing a solution containing 39 420 mg 2-propanol/litre water [56]. The germination of white amaranth (*Amaranthus albus*) seeds was not affected after 5 h of incubation at 25 °C on filter papers moistened with a solution containing 36 050 mg 2-propanol/litre of water [49]. Reynolds [216] measured 50% inhibition of germination in lettuce (*Lactuca sativa*) seeds after incubation for 3 days at 30 °C on agar containing 2100 mg 2-propanol/litre. At 6000 mg/litre, no germination at all was observed. However, above 18 030 mg/litre, germination was again observed and reached a maximum of 62% at 26 440 mg/litre. Inhibition of the growth of hypocotyls and rootlets after 6 days of incubation gradually increased with concentration. ED_{50} values were above 36 000 mg/litre.

In a 28-day study on cell suspensions of root sections of soybean, (*Glycine max*), at 26 °C and a pH of 5.6, onset of growth was delayed for 1 and 2 weeks at 2-propanol concentrations of 10 000 and 20 000 mg/litre of nutrient medium, respectively [67].

8. EFFECTS ON EXPERIMENTAL ANIMALS AND *IN VITRO* TEST SYSTEMS

8.1 Single Exposures

8.1.1 Mortality

Available acute mortality data are summarized in Table 9. Except where otherwise indicated, the vehicle was water or saline solution. LD_{50} values for several animal species after oral administration vary between 4475 and 7990 mg/kg body weight. Using 14-day-old rats of both sexes, Kimura et al. [134] established an oral LD_{50} of 4396 mg/kg body weight for undiluted 2-propanol; this was not significantly different from that obtained for young male adults (4710 mg/kg body weight) or older male adults (5338 mg/kg body weight).

8.1.2 Signs of intoxication

Sprague-Dawley rats of both sexes, inhaling 2-propanol for 8 h at concentrations between 19 680 and 64 206 mg/m^3, showed severe irritation of the mucous membranes and depression of the central nervous system indicated by subsequent ataxia, prostration, and narcosis. These effects were concentration- and time-dependent. Rats surviving the narcosis recovered. Transient paralysis of the hind limbs was observed at levels between 49 200 and 54 120 mg/m^3. The rats died at and above 44 280 mg/m^3, usually within 2 days, with females dying earlier than males. All rats were autopsied, including survivors, 15 days after exposure. At non-lethal levels, congestion of the liver, lung, and spleen were observed, especially in males. At lethal levels, vacuolation of the liver, acute pneumonitis, and spleen oedema were found. These effects were most pronounced in survivors. At 51 660 mg/m^3, severe cytoplasmic degeneration of the liver and oedema of the lung and brain occurred in all rats [151]. Deep narcosis occurred in rats exposed through inhalation to 40 mg/litre for 2 h. Significant and lasting hypothermia was induced in Sprague-Dawley rats exposed for 4 h to vapour concentrations of 19 680 mg/m^3 or more [151].

Table 9. Lethality of 2-propanol

Species/strain	Sex	Route of exposure	Observation period	LD$_{50}$ (mg/kg body weight)	LC$_{50}$ (mg/m^3)	Reference
Rat	not reported	oral	3 days	5 280	-	[157]
Sherman rat	not reported	oral	14 days	5 480	-	[239]
Sprague-Dawley rat	male	oral	7 days	4 710	-	[134]
Rat	not reported	oral	14 days	5 500	-	[103]
Mouse	not reported	oral	14 days	4 475	-	[103]
Rabbit	not reported	oral	3 days	5 030	-	[157]
Rabbit	male,	oral	1 day	7 990		[190]
Dog	not	oral	3 days	4 830		[157]
Wistar rat	male	intravenous	5 days	1 088	-	[247]
H mouse	male	intravenous	5 days	1 580	-	[247]
H mouse	female	intravenous	not reported	1 860		[56]
Chinchilla rabbit	male, female	intravenous	5 days	1 184	-	[247]
Wistar rat	male	intraperitoneal	5 days	2 830	-	[247]
H mouse	male	intraperitoneal	5 days	4 868	-	[247]
Syrian hamster	male	intraperitoneal	5 days	3 467	-	[247]
Rabbit	not reported	dermal	not reported	12 870		[239]
Rat	not reported	inhalation (4 h)	14 days	-	72 600	[103]
Sprague-Dawley rat	male	inhalation (8 h)	15 days	-	46 740	[150]
Sprague-Dawley rat	female	inhalation (8 h)	15 days	-	55 350	[150]
Mouse	not reported	inhalation (2 h)	14 days	-	53 000	[103]

Rats and mice of unknown strains, exposed orally or through inhalation to lethal levels of 2-propanol, showed unspecified signs of irritation and died through respiratory arrest while under narcosis, usually within 24 h following exposure. Necropsy revealed oedema, haemorrhage, inflammation, and dystrophy in the interstitial tissues of parenchymal organs. In the lung, infiltration, oedema, and thinning of the alveolar walls were observed [103].

The effects of 2-propanol on the mucociliary system of the trachea [197] and the middle ear [198] were investigated in two separate studies. Groups of 20 or 24 Hartley guinea-pigs were exposed to 2-propanol vapour at measured concentrations of 0, 969, or 13 382 mg/m^3 for 24 consecutive hours. Four animals from each of the 3 groups were killed by decapitation at 12 h, 24 h, and 3, 7, and 14 days after the exposure period. A concentration-related deterioration of ciliary activity and mucosal degeneration were observed in both the trachea and in the middle ear. At the lower exposure level, the effects completely reversed within 2 weeks of exposure, but, at the higher exposure level, they did not.

2-Propanol can enter the trachea and deeper lung structures by aspiration through the oral and nasal cavities. Anaesthetized rats were made to inspire 110 or 140 mg of the compound in water, or 160 mg of the undiluted compound. Survivors were sacrificed 24 h later for lung examination. At the lower doses, 1 out of 10 rats in each group died. At the highest dose, 6 out of 10 rats died of cardiac or respiratory arrest. All controls survived. It was not reported whether the latter were sham-exposed or not. The average absolute lung weight in the high-dose group was increased by 75% [94].

8.1.3 Skin, eye, and respiratory tract irritation

In primary irritation patch tests on groups of 6 rabbits and 6 Hartley guinea-pigs, 0.5 ml of undiluted 2-propanol was applied to areas of clipped or abraded skin. No irritation was observed for up to 48 h after a 4-h exposure [194]. Erythema and changes in vascular permeability did not occur when the clipped skin of guinea-pigs was exposed for 2 min to discs of filter paper soaked in undiluted 2-propanol [240].

Marzulli & Ruggles [182] reported on an interlaboratory evaluation of the ocular irritancy of 2-propanol, according to Draize scores, in groups of 6 rabbits, 1–7 days after application of 0.1 ml of a 70% solution on the cornea. One day after exposure, mean Draize scores were approximately 0.6 for corneal opacity, 0.3 for iritis, 1.5 for conjunctival redness, and 1.3 for chemosis. The maximum total Draize score was 10.1. In each laboratory, 67–97% of the rabbits met the criteria for eye irritation, which decreased over time. In another Draize test, groups of 6–9 New Zealand rabbits received doses of 70% 2-propanol at levels of 0.01, 0.03, or 0.10 ml per eye. Maximum total Draize scores were 21, 36, and 37, respectively, the maximum on the Draize scale being 110. Using irritation categories based on the number of days required for the effects to disappear, the compound was substantially irritating (clearing within 14 days) at the higher doses and moderately irritating (clearing within 7 days) at the lowest dose [100].

The eye irritancy of 2-propanol was evaluated using Stauffland albino rabbits, each of which received 0.1 ml of undiluted propanol in one eye. Eye irritation was scored according to Draize up to 21 days after application. The exact scores were not reported, but 2-propanol was found to be corrosive according to the US EPA criteria used in 1981, implying corneal involvement and irritation or eye damage that persisted for more than 21 days after treatment [188].

2-Propanol was tested on several occasions in *in vitro* cytotoxicity assays and the results showed good agreement with those *in vivo* [29, 30, 213].

The potency of 2-propanol as a sensory irritant was evaluated, using a 50% reflex decrease in the respiratory rate of mice (RD_{50}) as an index. The mice were exposed by their heads only. An exposure-related effect was found with RD_{50} values of 12 300 mg/m^3 for Swiss OF$_1$ mice and 43 525 mg/m^3 for Swiss Webster mice [61, 130].

8.2 Continuous or Repeated Exposures

Groups of rats were exposed to 2-propanol vapour at concentrations of 0, 100, or 500 mg/m^3 air for 5 days/week and 4 h/day over 4 months [103]. Strain, sex, and group size were not given, but were presumably in accordance with CMEA standards. No deaths were reported. At the end of 4 months of exposure to 500 mg/m^3 air, growth was reduced significantly by 10% and the respiratory rate was increased by 22%. The white blood cell count was decreased at both exposure levels in an exposure-related manner. At 500 mg/m^3, this was attributed to a decreased absolute and relative number of lymphocytes. Decreases in hippuric acid excretion and in total serum protein, and an increase in blood acetylcholine were found at both exposure levels. The decrease in total serum protein was exposure-related and could partly be accounted for by the observed decrease in α_1- and α_2-globulins and in albumin at 500 mg/m^3. Blood glucose levels were decreased at 500 mg/m^3. Macroscopic and microscopic changes, observed at 500 mg/m^3, included irritant effects on the respiratory system, such as thinning of the alveolar walls, perivascular infiltration, pneumonia, and bronchitis. Dystrophic changes and perivascular cell reactions were seen in the liver. Follicular hyperplasia was observed in the spleen [103].

Another report described the continuous exposure of groups of 15 rats of unknown strain and sex to 2-propanol vapour at concentrations of 0, 0.6, 2.5, or 20 mg/m^3 air for 86 days. The data were not statistically analysed. No deaths were reported. At the highest exposure level, changes in the latency period of unconditional reaction and an increase in the number of fluorescent leukocytes were found. Effects reported at this exposure level included an increase in sulfobromophthalein retention and decreased blood levels of nucleic acids. Microscopy only revealed adverse effects at 20 mg/m^3 with liver dystrophy, degenerative changes in the cerebral cortex, and spleen hyperplasia [19].

These studies [19, 103] lack a number of essential details concerning the protocol, the effects observed, the incidence of these effects, and the statistical analysis.

A "coefficient of accumulation" (the ratio between cumulative LD$_{50}$ and single dose LD$_{50}$) reported for repeated oral exposure to 2-propanol was 4.0 in rats and 4.9 in mice [10].

Groups of 5 white rats of each sex and of unknown strain received drinking-water containing 2-propanol for 27 weeks. Average daily intakes were 0, 600, or 2300 mg/kg body weight for males and 0,

1000, or 3900 mg/kg body weight for females. Only males died: 2 at the lower dose and 3 at the higher dose. It was reported that extensive postmortem changes prevented an accurate diagnosis of the cause of death. At the end of the exposure period, all exposed females showed growth retardation. Males showed a slight decrease in growth initially but overtook the controls in body weight towards the end of the exposure period. No adverse effects were found on food intake, behaviour, and histopathology [157].

8.3 Neurotoxicity and Behavioural Effects

2-Propanol passes the blood–brain barrier twice as effectively as ethanol (section 6.2.1). The oral ED_{50} for narcosis in rabbits exposed to 2-propanol was 2280 mg/kg body weight, i.e., 2.5 times lower than that for ethanol [190]. The threshold of an acute effect on the CNS was observed in rats after a 4-h exposure at 1450 mg/m^3 using the method of flexor reflexes, the "summation threshold method" [10]. The intraperitoneal ED_{50} for loss of righting reflex in Swiss Webster mice, which was 164 mg/kg body weight, was 1.8 times lower than that for ethanol [169]. The threshold for the induction of ataxia in Sprague-Dawley rats following intraperitoneal exposure was 1106 mg/kg body weight [171]. In 2 tilted plane tests, the performance of rats decreased by an average of 30–40% after oral or intraperitoneal exposure to 2000 and 1800 mg/kg body weight, respectively [178, 270]. On a molar basis, 2-propanol was 2.7 times as intoxicating as ethanol [270]. When C57BL/6J or DBA/2J mice were exposed intraperitoneally to a single dose of 2-propanol at 3 dose levels, the former strain showed increased activity in the open field test at 392 mg/kg body weight, no effect on activity at 785 mg/kg body weight, and narcosis at 1570 mg/kg body weight. DBA/2J mice showed increased activity at the middle dose level and narcosis at the high dose level [243]. Wistar rats, inhaling 2-propanol at a concentration of 739 mg/m^3 for 6 h/day, 5 days/week, for up to 15 weeks, did not show any adverse effects in the open field test [224].

The depressive action of 2-propanol on the central nervous system was related by several investigators to interactions with neuronal membranes *in vitro* and *in vivo*. Lyon et al. [169] observed a high correlation between the narcotic potencies of aliphatic alcohols in mice and their ability to disorder brain synaptosomal plasma membrane *in vitro*, as measured by electron paramagnetic resonance, which was, in turn, related to membrane solubility. In Sprague-Dawley rats, no change in synaptosomal membrane fluidity was measured via *in vitro* registration of the fluorescence polarization of 1,6-diphenyl-1,3,5-hexatriene, 20 h after a single oral dose of 3000 mg/kg body weight. When 2-propanol was added subsequently, a change in membrane fluidity was observed. This effect was related to membrane solubility. The activity of synaptosomal Na^+/K^+-transporting adenosinetriphosphatase (EC 3.6.1.37) was increased both *in vitro* and *in vivo* [24].

Functional loss due to disruption of membrane integrity by 2-propanol was also observed *in vitro* by the blocking of the action potentials of sciatic nerves in the toad, *Bufo marinus* [214], and by the inhibition of membrane-bound guanylate cyclase (EC 4.6.1.2) in intact murine neuroblastoma N1E-115 cells [241]. It was also indicated by the interference of 2-propanol with the transport of Ca^{2+} ions across biological membranes, as shown, *in vitro*, by the inhibition of Ca^{2+} ion-induced contractions of guinea-pig ileum (Yashuda et al., 1976), and, *in vivo*, in rats by a decrease in regional brain Ca^{2+} ion levels, 30 min after one intraperitoneal dose of 2000 mg/kg body weight [221].

Several neurochemical parameters were measured in the brain or spinal cord axon of Wistar rats, inhaling 2-propanol at a concentration of 739 mg/m^3 air for 6 h/day, 5 days/week, over 5, 10, 16, or 21 weeks. In cerebellar homogenates, the activities of superoxide dismutase (EC 1.15.1.1) and azoreductase (EC 1.6.6.7) were decreased at weeks 16 and 21, but no effects were found on the activity of dihydrolipoamide dehydrogenase (EC 1.8.1.4). In cerebellar glial cells, the activity of acid proteinase (EC 3.4.21.1) was stimulated at weeks 5 and 10, while the glutathione concentration was unaffected at all times. In the spinal cord axon, the phosphate/cholesterol ratio of lipid was reduced by 25% [224].

8.4 Biochemical Effects

8.4.1 Effects on lipids in liver and blood

Oral administration of single doses of 3000 or 6000 mg 2-propanol/kg body weight to Wistar rats caused a reversible accumulation of triglycerides in the liver [21, 22, 23, 90]. At the 6000 mg/kg body weight dose, a slight fatty infiltration was observed histologically [90]. Observations that could explain this effect were increased hepatic uptake of palmitate [23], increased incorporation of palmitate into hepatic triglycerides, decreased hepatic palmitate oxidation, and, at a later stage of intoxication, interference with the synthesis and excretion of very dense lipoproteins [21, 22, 23].

Decreased palmitate oxidation was related to the observed increase in the hepatic b-hydroxybutyrate/acetoacetate ratio, implying a decrease in the intramitochondrial $NAD^+/NADH$ ratio [21, 23, 195]. Excess extramitochondrial reducing equivalents, indicated by an increased lactate/pyruvate ratio, was also observed *in vivo* [21] and *in vitro* [85]. However, all these changes in the redox state of the liver were very modest and therefore were not thought to be fully responsible for the fatty livers induced.

More significant seemed to be the observation that the incorporation of palmitate and glycerol into serum triglycerides and the incorporation of palmitate into serum and hepatic phospholipids were inhibited. This indicates an impaired secretion of lipoproteins, partly explained by the observed disturbance of the biosynthesis of phospholipids, and partly by the observed inhibition of hepatic protein synthesis [21, 22, 23]. Inhibition of hepatic protein synthesis, as shown by the synthesis of the marker enzymes ornithine decarboxylase (EC 4.1.1.17) and tyrosine aminotransferase (EC 2.6.1.5), was observed in hepatectomized rats following oral exposure to 2300 mg 2-propanol/kg body weight [205].

Acetone administration to rats up to a blood level comparable to that in 2-propanol-dosed rats only slightly increased the level of liver triglycerides; therefore acetone does not seem to play a major role in the induction of fatty liver by 2-propanol [22].

8.4.2 Effects on microsomal enzymes

Oral exposure of Sprague-Dawley rats to 390 mg 2-propanol/kg body weight, once or on 4 subsequent days, caused a slight but significant increase in the hepatic cytochrome P-450 content and a 2–3-fold increase in the activities of the microsomal liver enzymes (EC 1.14.14.1) aniline hydroxylase and 7-ethoxycoumarin O-deethylase, 18 h after exposure [255]. Direct activation of these enzymes does not offer a satisfactory explanation, as it was shown *in vitro* that 2-propanol is an inhibitor of several microsomal enzymes via an interaction with cytochrome P-450, which causes a change in the reverse Type I spectrum [8, 57, 222, 246, 254, 285]. It was therefore concluded that, as acetone also does not appear to be involved in aniline hydroxylase induction *in vivo*, 2-propanol induces one or more forms of cytochrome P-450 [255]. In young Sprague-Dawley rats, receiving 2-propanol once at a level of 1960 or 3140 mg/kg body weight and sacrificed 22–24 h later, the hepatic cytochrome P-450 content increased, as well as the activities of several nitrosamine *N*-demethylases, benzphetamine demethylase, ethylmorphine demethylase, *p*-nitroanisole demethylase, and 7-ethoxycoumarin-*O*-deethylase. A slight increase was observed in the activity of NADPH cytochrome c reductase (EC 1.6.2.4). Acetone appeared to play a role in this induction. From several lines of observations, it was concluded that the enhanced activity of nitrosodimethylamine *N*-demethylase was due to the induction of specific forms of P-450 isozymes and P-450-dependent enzymes [255].

In several earlier studies on rats, at comparable or higher oral doses, induction of microsomal liver enzymes was observed, including a slight induction of NADPH cytochrome c reductase, but no increase in hepatic cytochrome P-450 content [206, 207, 234]. Ueng et al. [255] explained the latter observation by suggesting that the species of cytochrome P-450 induced must be normally present in low concentrations, so that a several-fold increase in catalytic activity could be induced without markedly increasing the total content of the haemoprotein.

Sprague-Dawley rats were also exposed by inhalation to 2-propanol at concentrations of 490, 4920, or 19 680 mg/m^3 air for 6 days/week, 6 h/day over 2 weeks. In the liver and kidneys, the contents of cytochrome P-450 and cytochrome b5 were increased as well as the activity of NADPH cytochrome c reductase at 4920 and 19 680 mg/m^3. These effects were completely reversible in the liver of rats exposed at 19 680 mg/m^3 for 2 weeks and allowed to recover for 4 weeks. However, they persisted in the kidneys [290].

8.4.3 Other biochemical findings

Differential effects have been observed on the glutathione status of the liver following exposure of rats to 2-propanol. In Sprague-Dawley rats inhaling 2-propanol at a concentration of 4920 or 19 680 mg/m^3 for 6 days/week, 6 h/day, over 2 weeks, the reduced glutathione concentration in the liver and kidneys increased slightly while, at 19 680 mg/m^3, the activity of glutathione S-transferase (EC 2.5.1.18) increased by 13% in the liver only [290]. The glutathione level in the liver of Wistar rats that had received a single oral dose of 3110 mg 2-propanol/kg body weight was reduced 6 h following exposure, while there was a 10% increase in lipid peroxidation, as indicated by the formation of diene conjugates [264]. A homogenate of normal or regenerating rat liver did not show any increase in malondialdehyde production after incubation with 2-propanol [6].

The activity of hepatic and kidney alanine aminotransferase (EC 2.6.1.2) in rats was unchanged 18 h after exposure to 1 or 4 daily doses of 392 mg 2-propanol/kg body weight [255] or 4 h after exposure to a single dose of 2300 mg/kg body weight [205]. Liver damage was not observed in guinea-pigs histopathologically or by any increase in serum ornithine carbamoyltransferase (EC 2.1.3.3), 24 h after receiving intraperitoneal doses of up to 1000 mg 2-propanol/kg body weight [73].

In Charles River rats, 2-propanol (785 mg/kg body weight ip) induced hepatic metallothionein and caused low blood zinc levels [244]. These changes were not prevented by adrenalectomy.

8.5 Immunological Effects

2-Propanol and acetone both enhanced the incorporation of labelled thymidine into concanavalin A-stimulated murine spleen cells *in vitro* [210]. 2-Propanol inhibited the killing of YAC-1 tumour cells by natural killer effector cells from mouse or rat spleens [219]. Inhibition of the synthesis and/or the secretion and/or function of at least one monocyte-derived substance that inhibited cell proliferation was suggested as an explanation of these findings [210].

8.6 Reproduction, Embryotoxicity, and Teratogenicity

Groups of 13–15 pregnant Sprague-Dawley rats were exposed to 2-propanol for 7 h/day on gestation days 1–19 at measured concentrations of 9001, 18 327, or 23 210 mg/m^3 (3659, 7450, or 9435 ppm). At the highest concentration, rats were completely narcotized at the end of the first exposures, but by the end of the 19 days the effect was slight. Initial exposures to 18 327 mg/m^3 (7450 ppm) caused an unsteady gait, but this was not noticeable by the end of 19 days of exposure. Food consumption and maternal body weight gain were significantly reduced by exposure to 18 327 and 23 210 mg/m^3 (7450 and 9435 ppm). In the group exposed to 23 210 mg/m^3 (9435 ppm): 6 out of 15 mated rats were not pregnant at term, which was attributed to an exposure-induced failure of implantation; 4 out of 9 pregnancies were totally resorbed; and resorptions per litter were significantly increased. Fetal body weights were significantly reduced, in a concentration-related pattern, at all 3 concentrations. The incidence of cervical ribs was significantly increased in the 23 210 mg/m^3 (9435 ppm) group [193].

A group of 6 female and 3 male rats (38–40 days old), of unspecified strain, received drinking-water containing 2-propanol. They were mated after approximately 2 months of exposure. This schedule was repeated through 2 further generations. Average daily intakes for the 3 generations were 1470, 1380, and 1290 mg/kg body weight, respectively. The growth of the first generation was retarded initially, but returned to normal by the 13th week. Otherwise, no effects were found on growth and reproductive functions [159].

When female hybrid rats received oral doses of 252 or 1008 mg 2-propanol/kg body weight per day for 45 days, the length of the estrus cycle was increased by 23–24% [15]. Five female hybrid rats also received daily doses of 1800 mg/kg body weight for 3 months before mating. Together with 6 controls they were sacrificed on day 21 of pregnancy. The total embryonic mortality rate was increased 2-fold, which was statistically significant [15].

In a 6-month drinking-water study, 2-propanol was administered to hybrid rats of both sexes, at daily doses of 0.018, 0.18, 1.8, or 18 mg/kg body weight. Mating of males with 5–7 females per group occurred after the exposure period. When both sexes were exposed to 18 mg/kg body weight, the litter size was increased. The neonatal mortality rate was increased at 0.18 and 1.8 mg/kg, when females only were exposed, at 18 mg/kg body weight, when males only were exposed, and at the 2 highest exposure levels, when both sexes were exposed. Neonates from the last group showed a dose-related decrease in the rate of reaction to electric stimuli (unconditioned defence reaction), but no other effects on their development [15].

Groups of 10–13 female hybrid rats received 252 or 1008 mg 2-propanol/kg body weight from day 1 to day 20 of pregnancy. They were sacrificed on day 21 of pregnancy together with 11 controls. Litter size was reduced at both exposure levels. General embryonic toxicity was 18 and 31%, respectively (10% in controls). At 1008 mg/kg body weight, total embryonic mortality rate was trebled and 10 out of 70 fetuses showed developmental anomalies compared with none out of 90 controls. The anomalies found were brain damage in 3 fetuses, kidney damage in 5 fetuses, and gastrointestinal damage in 2 fetuses. The lesions were not specified further. Data on maternal toxicity were not reported [15].

8.7 Mutagenicity

A reverse mutation spot test with the *Salmonella typhimurium* strains TA 98, TA 100, TA 1525, and TA 1537 was negative at 0.18 mg per plate, with and without metabolic activation by S9 rat liver [82].

Rat bone marrow cells were examined after 4 months of exposure of rats to 2-propanol vapour at concentrations of 0, 1.03, or 10.2 mg/m^3 air for 4 h/day. Statistically significant increases were counted in the percentage of mitotic aberrations [18]. However, the authors did not report the number of rats exposed, their sex, or strain.

Root tip cells of onion (*Allium cepa*) exposed to 2-propanol showed a 2.8-fold increase in the mitotic aberration rate [230].

2-Propanol did not increase sister chromatid exchange frequencies *in vitro* in V79 Chinese hamster lung fibroblasts, with or without S9 mix, when tested at concentrations of 3.3, 10, 33.3, and 100 mmol/ litre [267].

A dose-related increase in the inhibition of metabolic cooperation in hamster V79 cells, a phenomenon believed to reflect carcinogenic promotion ability and not to be indicative of genotoxic potential, was observed by Chen et al. [53]. This may be due to the membrane effects of 2-propanol.

8.8 Carcinogenicity

Several limited carcinogenicity studies on the mouse have been conducted with 2-propanol, using the inhalation, dermal, and subcutaneous routes of exposure.

Groups of 3 month-old, male C3H, ABC, and C57/BL mice were exposed to 2-propanol vapour at a concentration of 7700 mg/m^3 air for 3–7 h/day, 5 days/week, over 5–8 months. The sizes of the experimental and control groups were not reported. The occurrence of lung tumours was examined microscopically in mice that had survived until killed at the age of 8 months (36 exposed and 69 control C3H mice, 49 exposed and 120 control ABC mice), or 12 months (47 exposed and 52 control C57/BL mice) and showed macroscopic lesions. The mice were not examined for the occurrence of sinus tumours as occurred in workers engaged in the manufacture of 2-propanol (section 9.2.1). No excess of lung tumours was observed [276].

2-Propanol was painted on the clipped backs of 30 Rockland mice, 3 times/week for 1 year. Sex, dose, and observation period were not specified. Skin papillomas developed in 3 control mice, one of which also had a skin carcinoma, while there was no response in treated mice (Weil, C.S., written communication to US NIOSH [257]).

Groups of 3-month-old male C3H, ABC, and C57/BL mice received 20 mg undiluted 2-propanol subcutaneously once a week, for 20–40 weeks. The sizes of the treated and untreated control groups were not reported. Surviving mice that showed macroscopic lung lesions were examined microscopically for lung tumours. No excess of lung tumours was observed. Lung tumour incidence in the control group was high [276].

Doses of 20 mg undiluted 2-propanol were injected subcutaneously in 40 C3H mice, once a week, over a period of 20 weeks. Controls were untreated. The occurrence of lung tumours was examined in mice that survived until killed 5 months after the first injection (22 exposed and 33 control mice). No excess of lung tumours was observed (Weil, C.S., written communication to US NIOSH [257]).

In these studies, only lung tumours and, in the case of dermal exposure, skin tumours were investigated. Moreover, the exposure periods, where given, were too short to allow for tumour induction. Experimental details including size of experimental and control groups, sex ratio, and observation periods were not quoted for some of the studies. Because of these shortcomings, the studies are inadequate for the assessment of carcinogenic potential.

8.9 Factors Modifying Toxicity

As a result of the induction of specific isozymes of cytochrome P-450 (section 8.4.2) by 2-propanol and/or acetone, the hepatotoxicity of carbon tetrachloride, 1,1,2-trichloroethane, chloroform ($CHCl_3$), trichloroethylene, and dimethylnitrosamine in rodents is enhanced [60, 165, 234, 252, 253, 254]. The metabolic activation of n-hexane by liver and kidney microsomes is also increased by 2-propanol pretreatment [290].

9. EFFECTS ON MAN

9.1 General Population Exposure

9.1.1 Poisoning incidents

The subject of non-beverage alcohol use has already been addressed in section 5.2.2. The clinical literature has been reviewed [149, 176, 245, 163]. A brief summary of cases of intoxication and major symptoms is presented in Table 10.

Intoxications have been reported after oral ingestion (Table 10), rectal administration [59], and inhalation by children who have been sponged for several hours with 2-propanol preparations for fever reduction (Table 10). Skin absorption in 2-propanol sponging has been deemed insignificant [e.g., 149, 176]. However, a case report on a child with an almost lethal blood level of 2-propanol after sponge bathing for fever reduction, and questionable ingestion, suggested to the authors that the importance of dermal absorption, compared with inhalation, should not be underestimated [181].

2-Propanol depresses the central nervous system. At comparable doses, 2-propanol is thought to be approximately twice as active as ethanol in this respect with a longer duration of the coma due to slower metabolism and to the contribution of acetone to the depression of the central nervous system [149, 163, 176, 245]. As with ethanol, excessive intoxication with 2-propanol causes unconsciousness, usually, but not always ending in a deep coma [5, 59, 108, 128]; death may follow due to respiratory depression [4]. In most cases, decreased or absent reflexes are reported. Pupil size is variable, but most often miotic [16, 88, 149, 220, 228, 266]. Early gastrointestinal problems and hypothermia frequently occur. Cardiovascular effects include severe hypotension, shock [4, 266], and even cardiac arrest [176, 266]. Tachycardia is found as a secondary effect. Other possible compound-related effects are hyperglycaemia, elevated protein levels in cerebrospinal fluid [5, 170, 266], and atelectasis [191, 220]. Lung congestion was observed in fatal cases [4, 11].

Table 10. Acute intoxications by 2-propanol[a]

No. of cases	No. of alco- holics	Observations[b]							Reference
		1	2	3	4	5	6	7	
Ingestion									
57	46	+57							[11]
5	2	+5	+5	+4	+2	+4	+2		[4]
1[c]	0	-	+	+	+	+	+	+	[186]
3	3	-	+3	-	+2	+2	+1	+2	[170]
1	0	-	+	+	+	+	+	-	[191]
2	0	-	+2	+2		+2		+1	[149]
1	1	-	+	+	-	+	-	+	[245]
17	14	-	+2	+3	+10	-	-		[131]
1		-	+	+	+			-	[88]
1	1	-	+	+		+			[135]
1[c]	0	-	+	+	-	+	-	-	[266]
1	1	-	+	+	-		-	+	[261]
1	0	-	+				+		[75]
1	0	-	+		-		-	-	[220]
2	1	-	-	+	+2	-	+2	+1	[5]
1	1	-	-	-	+	-	+	-	[128]
1	1	-	-	-	+		+		[108]
Sponging									
1[c]	-	-	+	+	+	+	+		[228]
1[c]	-	-	+	+	+	-	-	+	[160]
1[c]	-	-	+		+		+		[91]
1[c]	-	-	+		+	-	-	+	[172]
1[c]	-	-	+						[181]
1[c]	-	-	+	+	+	+	-	+	[16]

[a] +N = observed in N cases; - = not observed; no sign = not reported.
[b] 1 = death;
  2 = coma;
  3 = hypotension, meaning ≤ 100 mm Hg systolic pressure and/or ≤ 60 mmHg diastolic pressure;
  4 = tachycardia, meaning ≥ 100 beats per min;
  5 = hypothermia, meaning ≤ 36.5 °C;
  6 = gastritis, characterized by nausea, vomiting, abdominal pain, and/or gastric haemorrhage;
  7 = elevated blood glucose, meaning ≥ 1500 mg/litre.

c Child below 2.5 years of age.

Effects on man

In cases of 2-propanol intoxication, hypotension can be a grave prognostic sign [4], which some authors suggest requires immediate action by gastric lavage, haemodialysis [5, 22, 88, 135, 176], or peritoneal dialysis [75, 186, 245]. Following treatment, recovery is usually complete, unless the hypotension is severe and persistent. In such cases, renal injury and death may occur [4, 128].

Acetone can be detected in the blood, urine, and breath. Because other ketone bodies are not found in significant quantities, early acidosis does not usually occur, serum bicarbonate, anion gap, and blood pH remaining normal. Sometimes, a mild metabolic acidosis and anion gap may develop as a result of lactic acid accumulation. Acetonaemia and/or acetonuria without metabolic acidosis and with normal or slightly elevated blood glucose levels differentiate 2-propanol poisoning from diabetic ketoacidosis and poisoning by other alcohols [16, 163, 176]. In addition, a significant osmolality gap may be observed [16, 261].

None of the biochemical findings could be related to blood levels of 2-propanol or acetone. 2-Propanol levels, measured at different times after exposure, varied between undetectable concentrations and 5600 mg/litre [176]. Acetone levels varied between undetectable concentrations and 18 780 mg/litre [75]. Alexander et al. [11] suggested that combined levels of 2-propanol and acetone may allow greater accuracy in predicting the clinical course of the condition of a patient.

Adults have been reported to survive ingestion of 700 ml of 2-propanol [88] and to die after ingestion of 400 ml of 2-propanol [4]. The lowest dose reported to be life-threatening was in an 18-month-old child who ingested approximately 170 ml of 2-propanol [186].

9.1.2 Controlled exposures

No adverse effects were observed in groups of 8 healthy male volunteers (24–57 years of age) who drank a daily dose of 2.6 or 6.4 mg 2-propanol/kg body weight in diluted syrup for 6 weeks. Investigations included haematology, blood chemistry, urinalysis, and ophthalmoscopy [283].

Another group of 10 healthy male volunteers (age not stated) was exposed to 2-propanol vapour at nominal concentrations of 490, 980, or 1970 mg/m^3 air for 3–5 min. After each exposure, the participants were asked to classify the effects of the vapour on the eyes, nose, and throat. The volunteers judged irritation to be "mild" at 980 mg/m^3 and "not severe" at 1970 mg/m^3. They also judged 490 mg/m^3 to be "satisfactory" for their own 8-h occupational exposure [192]. The validity of these results is doubtful, for various reasons including the subjective criteria used, the lack of control exposures, and the unreliability of the exposure levels.

9.1.3 Skin irritation; sensitization

No skin irritation was observed in 6 human volunteers when 0.5 ml of undiluted 2-propanol was applied to a 4 cm square area on the back and evaluated after 4 h, 24 h and 48 h [194]. Closed patch tests with 10-min applications of 0.1–0.3 ml undiluted 2-propanol on the dry skin of 10 healthy volunteers and 12 persons receiving disulfiram therapy for the treatment of chronic alcoholism did not result in any reaction. After immersion of the skin in tepid water for 10 min, a transient erythema rapidly appeared on the site of application in 19 subjects [105].

Skin irritation was also reported in a total of 6 premature infants with a gestational age of less than 27 weeks. They were exposed via swabs used for conduction in ECG recording or by the application of 2-propanol on the umbilical area with subsequent soaking of the diaper. Erythema and second or third degree burns or blisters were observed in areas of prolonged contact with 2-propanol. Hypoperfusion of the skin was suggested to be a contributing factor [226, 277].

In 1968, Wasilewski [272] reported a case of alleged allergic contact dermatitis following skin disinfection with a 70% 2-propanol swab. The patient was treated for allergic rhinitis. Patch tests were positive for 2-propanol. However, controls were not tested and there was no information on the purity of the alcohol. This report was followed by several others concerning a total of 8 persons who showed dermatitis after contact with medi-swabs containing 2-propanol. Patch testing revealed that another volatile agent, presumably propylene oxide, caused the effect [174, 124, 217]. Only one of these 8 persons was also hypersensitive to 2-propanol of unknown purity [124].

Itching eczematous lesions developed in a laboratory worker, in a company manufacturing hair cosmetics, in patch tests with chemically pure 2-propanol solutions (2.5–99.7% by volume). This person also reacted to 1-propanol, 1-butanol, 2-butanol, and formaldehyde, but not to ethanol and methanol. Controls were not tested [167]. Two out of 4 confirmed cases of hypersensitivity to primary alcohols were also found to be hypersensitive to secondary alcohols. Both cases had a history of contact allergies. Recurrent exposures to 2-propanol and/or other alcohols occurred through consumption of alcoholic beverages, pre-injection disinfection, via a hair lotion in one case and occupationally in the other case. Patch tests were positive for pure undiluted 2-propanol and 2-butanol. Twenty controls did not show any reactions to secondary alcohols [86, 87]. The mechanism of alcohol hypersensitivity is not clear. Fregert et al. [87] pointed out that it is difficult to understand how alcohols can act as haptens.

9.2 Occupational Exposure

9.2.1 Epidemiology studies

A retrospective cohort study was reported among 182 workers at a plant, in the USA, manufacturing 2-propanol by the strong acid process over the period 1928–50. In a subgroup of 71 men, who had been employed for more than 5 years, 7 cases of cancer were observed: 4 cancers of the paranasal sinuses, 1 lung carcinoma, 1 laryngeal carcinoma, and 1 laryngeal papilloma. The minimum latency period was 6 years [276]. According to USA vital statistics for 1948, 0.0014 paranasal sinus cancers would have been expected for the total cohort [286].

Two cases of paranasal sinus cancer and 2 cases of laryngeal cancer were reported in 1966 in a cohort of 779 workers in a similar plant in the USA that had been in operation since 1927. The minimum latency period was 10 years. The age- and sex-adjusted incidence of sinus and laryngeal cancer in this group was 21 times higher than expected [119].

Another retrospective cohort study was undertaken among 262 men who had worked for at least one year in a 2-propanol-manufacturing plant in the United Kingdom using the strong acid procedure over the period 1949–76. There were more than 4000 person-years at risk. No person was lost to follow-up, which was over an average of 15.5 years. The mortality rates due to all causes and due to neoplasms were not significantly higher than expected according to national vital statistics. One person died from nasal cancer against 0.02 expected. Other significant findings were 2 "kidney and adrenal malignancies" and 2 cancers of "the brain and the central nervous system" [9].

A fourth retrospective cohort study was conducted over the years 1966–78 among 433 workers in a 2-propanol manufacturing plant, in the USA, who were exposed for at least 3 months during the period 1941–65. The strong acid process used in 1941 had been gradually changed to the weak acid process by 1965. More than 11 000 person-years were at risk. The mortality rate due to all causes was lower than expected on the basis of state vital statistics. No excess mortality due to all cancers was observed, but the incidence of buccal and pharyngeal cancer was 4 times higher than expected (2 versus 0.5). There was a slight excess of lung cancer (7 versus 5.94) [79].

These cohort studies collectively suggest a cancer hazard related to the strong acid manufacturing process. The excess in respiratory cancers was initially attributed to isopropyl oils [119, 276]. However, the experimental basis for this assumption is weak (section 8.8) and more recently diisopropyl sulfate, an intermediate produced in the strong acid process, has been proposed as a more likely causative agent. The concentration of this chemical is high in the strong acid process and low in the weak acid process [79, 286].

Two small case-control studies were conducted in the USA: one to consider the risk of lymphocytic leukaemia associated with 24 solvents among rubber industry workers [52], and the other to consider the risk of brain gliomas associated with exposure conditions during work at a chemical plant [155]. Although there was no evidence of an association between exposure to 2-propanol and the incidence of gliomas or lymphocytic leukaemia, the small number of subjects and multiple exposures mean that no conclusions can be drawn from these studies.

9.2.2 Interacting agents

Fourteen out of 43 workers in a 2-propanol-packaging plant became ill when carbon tetrachloride was used for cleaning equipment. The incidence and the severity of the effects increased where exposure to carbon tetrachloride was the highest, and where, on another occasion, the mean concentration of 2-propanol in air was also highest, i.e., 1010 mg/m^3. In 4 cases, renal failure or hepatitis developed [83]. Another similar incident was reported in a colour printing factory, 17 workers had abnormal liver function and 3 developed acute hepatitis following combined exposure to carbon tetrachloride and 2-propanol [71]. These reports suggest potentiation of the toxicity of carbon tetrachloride by 2-propanol, which was also found in experimental animals (section 8.9).

Some shaving lotions containing 2-propanol and other ingredients (e.g., menthol, camphor, methyl salicylate, naphthalene) have been reported to produce central stimulation with motor restlessness, extreme apprehension, hallucinations, and general disorientation [89, 238].

10. EVALUATION OF HUMAN HEALTH RISKS AND EFFECTS ON THE ENVIRONMENT

10.1 Evaluation of Human Health Risks

10.1.1 Exposure

Exposure of human beings to 2-propanol may occur through inhalation during manufacture, processing, and both occupational and household use. Average concentrations of up to 35 mg/m^3 in the ambient urban air and up to 500 mg/m^3 in the occupational environment have been measured. Concentrations between 0.2 and 325 mg/litre have been found in non-alcoholic beverages, and between 50 and 3000 mg/kg in foods (section 5).

Exposure of the general public to a potentially lethal level may result from accidental or intentional ingestion and children may be exposed when sponged with 2-propanol preparations (rubbing alcohol) (sections 6 and 9).

10.1.2 Health effects

2-Propanol is rapidly absorbed after inhalation or ingestion and distributed throughout the body as such, sulfated, or as its metabolite, acetone (section 6). The possibility of dermal absorption should not be neglected.

The acute toxicity of 2-propanol for animals is low (based on lethality estimates) whether exposure occurs via the dermal, oral, or respiratory route.

In man, the most likely acute effects of exposure to high levels of 2-propanol by ingestion or inhalation are alcoholic intoxication and narcosis. The results of animal studies indicate that 2-propanol is approximately twice as intoxicating as ethanol with an oral ED$_{50}$ for rabbits of 2280 mg/kg and a threshold for ataxia in rats of 1106 mg/kg intraperitoneally (section 8.3). Oral LD$_{50}$ values in various species vary between 4475 and 7990 mg/kg and inhalation LC$_{50}$ values between 50 000 and 70 000 mg/m^3 (section 8.1.1).

Evaluation

Because ethanol retards the elimination of 2-propanol and is also a CNS depressant, interaction between ethanol and propanol may be expected to increase the CNS effects of either agent. The majority of acute intoxication cases involved ingestion by known alcoholics. Febrile children have experienced life-threatening intoxications when treated by skin sponging with 2-propanol. In these cases, skin absorption may also be an important route of exposure in addition to inhalation (section 9.1.1).

Exposure–effect data on human beings in an acute overexposure situation are scarce and show great variation. The major effects are gastritis, depression of the central nervous system with hypothermia and respiratory depression, and hypotension (section 9.1.1).

In rabbits, 2-propanol did not irritate the skin but did irritate the eyes when 0.1 ml undiluted compound was applied (section 8.1.3). Care is required in the use of 2-propanol as a disinfectant on premature babies as it may cause severe skin irritation following prolonged contact.

No adequate animal studies are available to make an evaluation of the human health risks associated with repeated exposure to 2-propanol. However, 2 studies in rats with inhalation (500 mg/m^3, 4 h/day, 5 days per week, for 4 months) or oral (600–3900 mg/kg in drinking-water) exposure suggest that exposure to 2-propanol at some of the very high occupational exposures reported should be avoided (section 8.2).

2-Propanol administered in the drinking-water has been tested for reproductive effects in a number of studies with conflicting results. In one study, impaired neonatal survival was reported after 6 months exposure of female rats to 0.18 mg/kg per day. In a multi-generation study there were no adverse effects at drinking-water doses as high as 1470 mg/kg per day. In a teratology study, drinking-water doses of 252 and 1008 mg/kg per day produced developmental toxicity, but this was not related to maternal toxicity. Inhalation exposure of pregnant rats to 2-propanol provided a LOEL of 18 327 mg/m^3 (7450 ppm) and a NOEL of 9001 mg/m^3 (3659 ppm) for maternal toxicity. In the same study, 9001 mg/m^3 (3659 ppm) was a LOEL for developmental toxicity, with no demonstration of a NOEL (section 8.6). These concentrations are higher than those likely to be encountered under conditions of human exposure.

2-Propanol was negative in a bacterial spot test and in a test for sister chromatid exchange in mammalian cells *in vitro*. It induced mitotic aberrations in the bone marrow of rats. Although these findings suggest that the substance has no genotoxic potential, no adequate assessment of mutagenicity can be made on the basis of the limited data available. An *in vitro* test said to predict promotional activity was negative (section 8.7).

The data available are inadequate to assess the carcinogenicity of 2-propanol in experimental animals (section 8.8). There are no data to assess the carcinogenicity of 2-propanol itself in human beings. There are adequate data to indicate that the strong acid process for the production of 2-propanol is causally associated with the induction of paranasal sinus cancer in human beings, probably due to exposure to the intermediate, di-2-propyl sulfate, an alkylating agent and not to 2-propanol itself (section 9.2.1).

2-Propanol is shown to potentiate the hepatic toxicity of halocarbons, such as carbon tetrachloride. Therefore simultaneous exposure to 2-propanol and halocarbons should be avoided (section 9.2.2).

The Task Group considers it unlikely that 2-propanol will pose a serious health risk to the general population under exposure conditions likely to be encountered.

10.2 Evaluation of Effects on the Environment

By reacting with hydroxyl radicals and through rain-out, 2-propanol will disappear rapidly from the atmosphere, with a residence time of less than 2.5 days (section 4.2). Hydrolysis and photolysis are not important in the removal of 2-propanol from water and soil but removal occurs quite rapidly by aerobic and anaerobic biodegradation, especially after adaptation of initially seeded microorganisms (section 4.3.1). Adsorption of 2-propanol on soil particles is poor but it should be mobile in soil and it has been shown to increase the permeability of soil to some aromatic hydrocarbons.

In view of the physical properties of 2-propanol, its potential for bioaccumulation is low (section 4.3.2).

Toxicity in aquatic organisms was observed at levels ranging from 104 mg/litre for one protozoan to over 50 000 mg/litre for Tubifex worms. Insects and plant seeds were only affected at concentrations above 2000 mg/litre (section 7).

On the basis of these data, it can be concluded that, except in cases of accident and inappropriate disposal, 2-propanol does not present a risk to naturally occurring organisms at concentrations that usually occur in the environment.

11. RECOMMENDATIONS

1. 2-Propanol has not shown mutagenic potential in the small number of assays performed. A full array of modern genotoxicity tests should be completed.

2. Several studies of the carcinogenic activity of 2-propanol have been published but all are seriously flawed and cannot be used to evaluate the potential carcinogenicity of 2-propanol. The desirability of a carcinogenesis bioassay of 2-propanol should be considered based on the outcome of genotoxicity tests.

3. Inhalation exposure to overtly toxic concentrations of 2-propanol produced reproductive and developmental toxicity. Additionally, the data available from drinking-water studies are conflicting. In view of the potential for environmental and drinking-water contamination, reproductive and developmental toxicity should be conducted using oral dosing.

4. Epidemiological studies including precise exposure data would assist in an assessment of the occupational hazards from 2-propanol.

12. PREVIOUS EVALUATIONS BY INTERNATIONAL BODIES

An evaluation of the carcinogenicity of 2-Propanol by the International Agency for Research on Cancer[a] was reported as follows:

"**A. Evidence for carcinogenicity to humans** (*sufficient for the manufacture of isopropyl alcohol by the strong-acid process; inadequate for isopropyl alcohol and isopropyl oils*).

An increased incidence of cancer of the paranasal sinuses was observed in workers at factories where isopropyl alcohol was manufactured by the strong-acid process. The risk for laryngeal cancer may also have been elevated in these workers. It is unclear whether the cancer risk is due to the presence of diisopropyl sulfate, which is an intermediate in the process, to isopropyl oils, which are formed as by-products, or to other factors, such as sulfuric acid. Epidemiological data concerning the manufacture of isopropyl alcohol by the weak-acid process are insufficient for an evaluation of carcinogenicity."

"**B. Evidence for carcinogenicity to animals** (*inadequate for isopropyl alcohol and isopropyl oils*).

Isopropyl oils, formed during the manufacture of isopropyl alcohol by both the strong-acid and weak-acid processes, were tested inadequately in mice by inhalation, skin application and subcutaneous administration. Isopropyl oils formed during the strong-acid process were also tested inadequately in dogs by inhalation and instillation into the sinuses.

The available data on isopropyl alcohol were inadequate for evaluation."

"**C. Other relevant data**

No data were available to the Working Group."

---

[a] International Agency for Research on Cancer, *Overall Evaluations of Carcinogenicity: An updating of IARC Monographs volumes 1 to 42.* Lyon, France, 1987 (IARC Monographs on the Evaluation of Carcinogenic Risks to Humans, Supplement 7)

REFERENCES

1. ABSHAGEN, U. & RIETBROCK, N. (1969) [Elimination of 2-propanol in dogs and rats.] *Naunyn-Schmiedebergs Arch. Pharmakol. exp. Pathol.*, **264**: 110-118 (in German).

2. ABSHAGEN, U. & RIETBROCK, N. (1970) [The mechanism of the 2-propanol oxidation.] *Naunyn-Schmiedebergs Arch. Pharmakol. exp. Pathol.*, **265**: 411-424 (in German).

3. ACKMAN, R.G., HINLEY, H.J., & POWER, H.E. (1967) Determination of isopropyl alcohol in fish protein concentrate by solvent extraction and gas-liquid chromatography. *J. Fish. Res. Board Can.*, **24**: 1521-1529.

4. ADELSON, L. (1962) Fatal intoxication with isopropyl alcohol (rubbing alcohol). *Am J. clin. Pathol.*, **38**: 144-151.

5. AGARWAL, S.K. (1979) Non-acidotic acetonemia: a syndrome due to isopropyl alcohol intoxication. *J. Med. Soc. New Jersey*, **76**: 914-916.

6. AGOSTINI, C. (1982) Effects of various inhibitors on lipid peroxidation by homogenates of normal, regenerating and hepatomous rat liver, by liver slices and by hepatoma cells. *Med. Biol. Environ.*, **10**: 3-15.

7. AHAMED, A. & MATCHES, J.R. (1983) Alcohol production by fish spoilage bacteria. *J. food Prot.*, **46**: 1055-1059.

8. AKHREM, A.A., POPOVA, E.M., & METELITSA, D.I. (1978) [Interaction of aliphatic alcohols with cytochrome P-450 from rat liver microsomes.] *Biokhimiya (Mosk)*, **43**: 1485-1491 (in Russian).

9. ALDERSON, M.R. & RATTAN, N.S. (1980) Mortality of workers on an isopropyl alcohol plant and two MEK dewaxing plants. *Br. J. ind. Med.*, **37**: 85-89.

10. ALEKPEROV, I.I. & GUSEINOV, V.G. (1980) *Toxicological characteristics of isopropanol as an industrial poison, All Union Foundation Conference on Toxicology, Moscow, 25-27 November 1980*, p. 33.

11 ALEXANDER, C.B., MCBAY, A.J., & HUDSON, R.P. (1982) Isopropanol and isopropanol deaths: ten years' experience. *J.. forensic Sci.*, **27**: 541-548.

12 ANDERS, M.W. & HARRIS, R.N. (1981) Effect of 2-propanol treatment on carbon tetrachloride metabolism and toxicity. *Adv. exp. Med. Biol.*, **136A**: 591-602.

References

13 ANDERSON, S.M. & MCDONALD, J.F. (1981) Effect of environmental alcohol on *in vivo* properties of *Drosophila* alcohol dehydrogenase. *Biochem. Genet.*, **19**: 421-430.

14 ANON. (1987) Chemical market profile: isopropanol. *Chem. Market. Rep.*, **31 August**: 46.

15 ANTONOVA, V.I. & SALMINA, Z.A. (1978) [The maximum permissible concentration of isopropyl alcohol in water bodies with due regard for its action on the gonads and the progeny.] *Gig. i Sanit.*, **43**: 8-11 (in Russian).

16 ARDITI, M. & KILLMER, M.S. (1987) Coma following use of rubbing alcohol for fever control. *Am. J. DC*, **141**: 237-238.

17 ARISTOV, V.N. (1982) [Combined effect of toluene, isopropanol, and sulfur dioxide in conditions of petrochemical production.] *Gig. Tr. Prof. Zabol.*, **ISS9**: 5-9 (in Russian).

18 ARISTOV, V.N., REDKIN, Y.V., BRUSKIN, Z.Z., & OGLEZNEV, G.A. (1981) [Experimental data on the mutagenous effects of toluene, isopropanol, and sulfur dioxide.] *Gig. Tr. Prof. Zabol.*, **25**: 33-36 (in Russian).

19 BAIKOV, B.K., GORLOVA, O.E., GUSEV, M.I., NOVIKOV, Y.V., YUDINA, T.V., & SERGEEV, A.N. (1974) [Hygienic standardization of the daily average maximal permissible concentrations of propyl and isopropyl alcohols in the atmosphere.] *Gig. i Sanit.*, **4**: 6-13 (in Russian).

20 BALD, E. & MAZURKIEWICZ, B. (1980) Analytical utility of 2-halopyridinium salts. Part III. Paper electrophoretic characterization of alcohols as 2-alkoxy-1-methylpyridinium *p*-toluenesulfonates. *Chromatographia*, **13**: 295-297.

21 BEAUGE, F., CLEMENT, M., RENAUD, G., NORDMANN, R., & NORDMANN, J. (1975) Action de l'isopropanol sur le métabolisme lipidique chez le rat: etudes complémentaires sur les mécanismes impliqués dans l'accumulation hépatique des triacylglycérides. *Arch. int. Physiol. Biochim.*, **83**: 573-591.

22 BEAUGE, F., CLEMENT, M., NORDMANN, J., & NORDMANN, R. (1977) Etudes comparatives des actions de l'acétone et de l'isopropanol sur le métabolisme lipidique chez le rat. *Arch. int. Physiol. Biochim.*, **85**: 931-940.

23 BEAUGE, F., CLEMENT, M., NORDMANN, J., & NORDMANN, R. (1979) Comparative effects of ethanol, *n*-propanol and isopropanol on lipid disposal by rat liver. *Chem.-biol. Interact.*, **26**: 155-166.

24 BEAUGE, F., FLEURET, C., BARIN, F., & NORDMANN, R. (1984) Brain membrane disordering after acute in vivo administration of ethanol, isopropanol or t-butanol in rats. Biochem. Pharmacol., **33**: 3591-3595.

25 BESS, F.D. & CONWAY, R.A. (1966) Aerated stabilization of synthetic organic chemical wastes. J.. Water Pollut. Control Fed., **38**: 939-956.

26 BLACKMAN, R.A.A. (1974) Toxicity of oil-sinking agents. Mar. Pollut. Bull., **5**: 116-118.

27 BONTE, W., RUDELL, E., SPRUNG, R., FRAUENRATH, C., BLANKE, E., KUPILAS, G., WOCHNIK, J. & ZAH, G. (1981a) [Experimental investigations concerning the analytical detection of small doses of higher aliphatic alcohols in blood in man.] Blutalkohol, **18**: 399-411 (in German).

28 BONTE, W., SPRUNG, R., RUDELL, E., FRAUENRATH, C., BLANKE, E., KUPILAS, G., WOCHNIK, J., & ZAH, G. (1981b) [Experimental investigations concerning the analytical detection of small doses of higher aliphatic alcohols in human urine.] Blutalkohol, **18**: 412-426 (in German).

29 BORENFREUND, E. & BORRERO, O. (1984) In vitro cytotoxicity assays. Potential alternatives to the Draize ocular allergy test. Cell Biol. Toxicol., **1**: 55-65.

30 BORENFREUND, E. & SHOPSIS, C. (1985) Toxicity monitored with a correlated set of cell-culture assays. Xenobiotica, **15**: 705-711.

31 BOSSET, J.O. & LIARDON, R. (1984) The aroma composition of Swiss Gruyere cheese. II. The neutral volatile components. Lebensm.-Wiss. Technol., **17**: 359-362.

32 BOUGHTON, L.L. (1944) The relative toxicity of ethyl and isopropyl alcohols as determined by long term rat feeding and external application. Am. pharm. Assoc., **33**: 111-113.

33 BRIDIE, A.L., WOLFF, C.J.M., & WINTER, M. (1979a) BOD and COD of some petrochemicals. Water Res., **13**: 627-630.

34 BRIDIE, A.L., WOLFF, C.J.M., & WINTER, M. (1979b) The acute toxicity of some petrochemicals to goldfish. Water Res., **13**: 623-626.

35 BRINGMANN, G. (1975) [Determination of the harmful biological action of water-endangering substances through inhibition of cell multiplication in the blue alga Microcystis.] Ges.-Ing., **96**: 238-241 (in German).

36 BRINGMANN, G. (1978) [Determination of the harmful biological action of water-endangering substances on protozoa. I. Bacteria fed flagellates.] Z. Wasser-Abwasser Forsch., **11**: 210-215 (in German).

References

37 BRINGMANN, G. & KUHN, R. (1977) [Limiting values of the harmful action of water-endangering substances on bacteria (*Pseudomonas putida*) and green algae (*Scenedesmus quadricauda*) in the cell multiplication inhibition test.] *Z. Wasser-Abwasser Forsch.*, **10**: 87-98 (in German).

38 BRINGMANN, G. & KUHN, R. (1980) [Determination of the harmful biological action of water-endangering substances on protozoa. II. Bacteria fed ciliates.] *Z. Wasser-Abwasser Forsch.*, **13**: 26-31 (in German).

39 BRINGMANN, G. & KUHN, R. (1982) [Findings regarding the harmful action of water-endangering substances on *Daphnia magna* in a further developed standardised test.] *Z. Wasser-Abwasser Forsch.*, **15**: 1-16 (in German).

40 BRINGMANN, G., KUHN, R. & WINTER, A. (1980) [Determination of the harmful biological action of water-endangering substances on protozoa. III. Saprozoic flagellates.] *Z. Wasser-Abwasser Forsch.*, **13**: 170-173 (in German).

41 BRUGNONE, F., PERBELLINI, L., APOSTOLI, P., BELLOMI, M., & CARETTA, D. (1983) Isopropanol exposure: environmental and biological monitoring in a printing works. *Br. J. ind. Med.*, **40**: 160-168.

42 BUFFONI, F., SANTONI, G., ALBANESE, V., & DOLARA, P. (1983) Urinary mercapturic acid in chemical workers and in control subjects. *J. appl. Toxicol.*, **3**: 63-65.

43 BULICH, A.A. (1979) Use of luminescent bacteria for determining toxicity in aquatic environments. In: Marking, L.L. & Kimerle, R.A., ed. *Aquatic toxicology*, American Society for Testing and Materials, pp. 98-106 (ASTM STP 667).

44 BULICH, A.A., GREENE, M.W., & ISENBERG, D.L. (1981) Reliability of the bacterial luminescence assay for determination of the toxicity of pure compounds and complex effluents. In: Branson, D.R. & Dickson, K.L., ed. *Aquatic toxicology and hazard assessment*. Fourth Conference, American Society for Testing and Materials, pp. 338-347 (ASTM STP 737).

45 CALHOUN, M.J. & DELLAMONICA, E.S. (1974) Determination of 2-propanol residue in some fruits dewaxed with alcohol vapors. *J. Assoc. Off. Anal. Chem.*, **57**: 1342-1345.

46 CARTER, W.P.L., DARNALL, K.R., GRAHAM, R.A., WINER, A.M., & PITTS, J.N. (1979) Reactions of C_2 and C_4 α-hydroxy radicals with oxygen. *J. phys. Chem.*, **83**: 2305-2311.

47 CEC (1982) Propan-2-ol: chemico-physical data, toxicity data, environmental occurrence, and permissible levels. In: *Report of the Scientific Committee for Food on Extraction Solvents*, Brussels, Belgium, Commission of the European Communities, Directorate General for Internal Market and Industrial Affairs, pp. 46-72.

48 CEDERBAUM, A.I., QURESHI, A., & MESSENGER, P. (1981) Oxidation of isopropanol by rat liver microsomes. Possible role of hydroxyl radicals. *Biochem. Pharmacol.*, **30**: 825-831.

49 CHADOEUF-HANNEL, R. & TAYLORSON, R.B. (1985) Anaesthetic stimulation of *Amaranthus albus* seed germination: interaction with phytochrome. *Physiol. Plant*, **65**: 451-454.

50 CHARBONNEAU, M., IJIMA, M., COTE, M.G., & PLAA, G.L. (1985) Temporal analysis of rat liver injury following potentiation of carbon tetrachloride hepatotoxicity with ketonic or ketogenic compounds. *Toxicology*, **35**: 95-112.

51 CHARRETON, M. (1981) Estimation des rejets de vapeurs de solvants au voisinage d'une usine de peintures. *Double Liaison - Chimie des Peintures*, **28**: 233-241.

52 CHECKOWAY, H., WILCOSKY, T., WOLF, P., & TYROLER, H. (1984) An evaluation of associations of leukemia and rubber industry solvent exposures. *Am. J. ind. Med.*, **5**: 239-249.

53 CHEN, T.-H., KAVANAGH, T.J., CHANG, C.C., & TROSKO, J.E. (1984) Inhibition of metabolic cooperation in Chinese hamster V79 cells by various organic solvents and simple compounds. *Cell Biol. Toxicol.*, **1**: 155-171.

54 CHEN, W.-S. & PLAPP, B.V. (1980) Kinetics and control of alcohol oxidation in rats. *Adv. exp. Med. Biol.*, **132**: 543-549.

55 CHOU, W.L., SPEECE, R.E., & SIDDIQI, R.H. (1978) Acclimation and degradation of petrochemical wastewater components by methane fermentation. *Biotechnol. Bioeng. Symp.*, **8**: 391-414.

56 CHVAPIL, M., ZAHRADNIK, R., & CMUCHALOVA, B. (1962) Influence of alcohols and potassium salts of xanthogenic acids on various biological objects. *Arch. int. Pharmacodyn. Ther.*, **135**: 330-343.

57 COHEN, G.M. & MANNERING, G.J. (1973) Involvement of a hydrophobic site in the inhibition of the microsomal p-hydroxylation of aniline by alcohols. *Mol. Pharmacol.*, **9**: 383-397.

58 COLEMAN, R.L., LUND, E.D., & SHAW, P.E. (1972) Analysis of grapefruit essence and aroma oils. *J. agric. food Chem.*, **20**: 100-103.

59 CORBETT, J. & MEIER, G. (1968) Suicide attempted by rectal administration of drug. *J. Am. Med. Assoc.*, **206**: 2320-2321.

60 CORNISH, H.H. & ADEFUIN, J. (1967) Potentiation of carbon tetrachloride toxicity by aliphatic alcohols. *Arch. environ. Health*, **14**: 447-449.

61 CUPITT, L.T. (1980) *Fate of toxic and hazardous materials in the air environment*, Research Triangle Park, North Carolina, US Environmental Protection Agency, Environmental Sciences Laboratory, Office of Research and Development (EPA 600/3-80-084, PB 80-221948).

62 CURTIS, C., LIMA, A., LOZANO, S.J., & VEITH, G.D. (1982) Evaluation of a bacterial bioluminiscence bioassay as a method for predicting acute toxicity of organic chemicals to fish. In: Pearson, J.G., Foster, R.B., & Bishop, W.E., ed. *Aquatic Toxicology and Hazard Assessment. Fifth Conference*, American Society for Testing and Materials, pp. 170-178 (ASTM STP 766).

63 DAINTY, R.H., EDWARDS, R.A., & HIBBARD, C.M. (1984) Volatile compounds associated with the aerobic growth of some *Pseudomonas* species on beef. *J. appl. Bacteriol.*, **57**: 75-81.

64 DALZIEL, K. & DICKINSON, F.M. (1966) The kinetics and mechanism of liver alcohol dehydrogenase with primary and secondary alcohols as substrates. *Biochem. J.*, **100**: 34-46.

65 DANIEL, D.R., MCANALLEY, B.H., & GARRIOTT, J.C. (1981) Isopropyl alcohol metabolism after acute intoxication in humans. *J. anal. Toxicol.*, **5**: 110-112.

66 DAVID, J. & BOCQUET, C. (1976) Compared toxicities of different alcohols for two *Drosophila* sibling species: *D. melanogaster* and *D. simulans*. *Comp. Biochem. Physiol.*, **54C**: 71-74.

67 DAVIS, D.G., WERGIN, W.P., & DUSBABEK, K.E. (1978) Effects of organic solvents on growth and ultrastructure of plant cell suspensions. *Pestic. Biochem. Physiol.*, **8**: 84-97.

68 DAVIS, P.L., DAL CORTIVO, L.A., & MATURO, J. (1984) Endogenous isopropanol: forensic and biochemical implications. *J. anal. Toxicol.*, **8**: 209-212.

69 DE CEAURRIZ, J.C., MICILLINO, J.C., BONNET, P., & GUENIER, J.P. (1981) Sensory irritation caused by various industrial airborne chemicals. *Toxicol. Lett.*, **9**: 137-143.

70 DEL ROSARIO, R., DE LUMEN, B.O., HABU, T., FLATH, R.A., MON, T.R., & TERANISHI, R. (1984) Comparison of headspace volatiles from winged beans and soybeans. *J. agric. food Chem.*, **32**: 1011-1015.

71 DENG, J.-F., WANG, J.-D., SHIH, T.-S., & LAN, F.-L. (1987) Outbreak of carbon tetrachloride poisoning in a color printing factory related to the use of isopropyl alcohol and an air conditioning system in Taiwan. *Am. J. ind. Med.*, **12**: 11-19.

72 DGEP (1987) *Review of literature data on 2-propanol*, Leidschendam, Netherlands, Directorate-General of Environmental Protection, Ministry of Housing, Physical Planning and Environment.

73 DIVINCENZO, G.D. & KRASAVAGE, W.J. (1974) Serum ornithine carbamyl transferase as a liver response test for exposure to organic solvents. *Am. Ind. Hyg. Assoc. J.*, **35**: 21-29.

74 DORIGAN, J., FULLER, B., & DUFFY, R. (1976) *Scoring of organic air pollutants. Chemistry, production and toxicity of selected synthetic organic chemicals*, The MITRE Corporation (MITRE Technical Report MTR-7248, Rev. 1, Appendix III).

75 DUA, S.L. (1974) Peritoneal dialysis for isopropyl alcohol poisoning. *J. Am. Med. Assoc.*, **230**: 35.

76 DUVEL, W.A. & HELFGOTT, T. (1975) Removal of wastewater organics by reverse osmosis. *J. Water Pollut. Control Fed.*, **47**: 57-65.

77 EGBERT, A.M., REED, J.S., POWELL, B.J., LISKOW, B.I., & LIESE, B.S. (1985) Alcoholics who drink mouthwash: the spectrum of nonbeverage alcohol use. *J. Stud. Alcohol*, **46**: 473-481.

78 EGOROV, Y.L. (1966) Vision of workers engaged in the production of synthetic fatty acids and issues relative to setting hygienic standards for the alcohol content in the air. *Gig. Tr. Prof. Zabol.*, **7**: 33-38.

79 ENTERLINE, P.E. (1982) Importance of sequential exposure in the production of epichlorohydrin and isopropanol. *Ann. N.Y. Acad. Sci.*, **381**: 344-349.

80 FANG, H.H.P & CHIAN, E.S.K. (1976) Reverse osmosis separation of polar organic compounds in aqueous solution. *Environ. Sci. Technol.*, **10**: 364-369.

81 FERNANDEZ, F. & QUIGLEY, R.M. (1985) Hydraulic conductivity of natural clays permeated with simple liquid hydrocarbons. *Can. Geotech. J.*, **22**: 205-214.

82 FLORIN, I., RUTBERG, L., CURVALL, M., & ENZELL, C.R. (1980) Screening of tobacco smoke constituents for mutagenicity using the Ames test. *Toxicology*, **18**: 219-232.

References

83 FOLLAND, D.S., SCHAFFNER, W., GINN, E., CROFFORD, O.B., & MCMURRAY, D.R. (1976) Carbon tetrachloride toxicity potentiated by isopropyl alcohol. Investigation of an industrial outbreak. *J. Am. Med. Assoc.*, **236**: 1853-1856.

84 FORE, S.P., RAYNER, E.T., & DUPUY, H.P. (1971) Determination of residual solvent in oilseed meals and flours. III. Isopropanol. *J. Am. Oil Chem. Soc.*, **48**: 140-142.

85 FORSANDER, O.A. (1967) Influence of some aliphatic alcohols on the metabolism of rat liver slices. *Biochem. J.*, **105**: 93-97.

86 FREGERT, S., GROTH, O., HJORTH, N., MAGNUSSON, B., RORSMAN, H., & OVRUM, P. (1969) Alcohol dermatitis. *Acta dermatovenereol.*, **49**: 493-497.

87 FREGERT, S., GROTH, O., GRUVBERGER, B., MAGNUSSON, B., MOBACKEN, H., & RORSMAN, H. (1971) Hypersensitivity to secondary alcohols. *Acta dermatovenereol.*, **51**: 271-272.

88 FREIREICH, A.W., CINQUE, T.J., XANTHAKY, G., & LANDAU, D. (1967) Hemodialysis for isopropanol poisoning. *New Engl. J. Med.*, **277**: 699-700.

89 GADSDEN, R.H., MELETTE, R.R., & MILLER, W.C. (1958) Scrap iron intoxication. *J. Am. Med. Assoc.*, **168**: 1220-1224.

90 GAILLARD, D. & DERACHE, R. (1966) Action de quelques alcools aliphatiques sur la mobilisation de différentes fractions lipidiques chez la rate. *Food cosmet. Toxicol.*, **4**: 515-520.

91 GARRISON, R.F. (1953) Acute poisoning from use of isopropyl alcohol in tepid sponging. *J. Am. Med. Assoc.*, **152**: 317-318.

92 GEORGE, H.A., JOHNSON, J.L., MOORE, W.E.C., HOLDEMAN, L.V., & CHEN, J.S. (1983) Acetone, isopropanol, and butanol production by *Clostridium beijerinckii* (syn. *Clostridium butylicum*) and *Clostridium aurantibutyricum*. *Appl. environ. Microbiol.*, **45**: 1160-1163.

93 GEORGE, V., SHARMA, S.D., TRIPATHI, A.K., & ABRAHAM, S.P. (1985) Flavour components of some edible fungi from Kashmir. I. *Pafai J.*, **7**: 27-30.

94 GERARDE, H.W., AHLSTROM, D.B., & LINDEN, N.J. (1966) The aspiration hazard and toxicity of a homologous series of alcohols. *Arch. environ. Health*, **13**: 457-461.

95 GERHOLD, R.M. & MALANEY, G.W. (1966) Structural determinants in the oxidation of aliphatic compounds by activated sludge. *J. Water Pollut. Control Fed.*, **38**: 562-579.

96 GILLETTE, L.A., MILLER, D.L., & REDMAN, H.E. (1952) Appraisal of a chemical waste problem by fish toxicity tests. *Sewage ind. Waste,* **24**: 1397-1401.

97 GIUSTI, D.M., CONWAY, R.A., & LAWSON, C.T. (1974) Activated carbon adsorption of petrochemicals. *J. Water Pollut. Control Fed.,* **46**: 947-965.

98 GORLOVA, O.E. (1970) [Hygienic assessment of isopropyl alcohol as an atmospheric pollutant.] *Gig. i Sanit.,* **35**: 9-14 (in Russian).

99 GOTZ-SCHMIDT, E.-M. & SCHREIER, P. (1986) Neutral volatiles from blended endive (*Cichorium endivia* L.). *J. agric. food Chem.,* **34**: 212-215.

100 GRIFFITH, J.F., NIXON, G.A., BRUCE, R.D., REER, P.J., & BANNAN, E.A. (1980) Dose-response studies with chemical irritants in the albino rabbit eye as a basis for selecting optimum testing conditions for predicting hazard to the human eye. *Toxicol. appl. Pharmacol.,* **55**: 501-513.

101 GUNTER, B. (1982)*Health hazard evaluation: Jeppesen Sanderson Inc.,* Cincinnati, Ohio, US National Institute for Occupational Safety and Health (HETA 81-261-1085, PB 83-201749).

102 GUNTER, B.J., LIGO, R.L., & RUHE, R.L. (1976) *Health hazard evaluation determination, Steiger Tractor Inc.,* Cincinnati, Ohio, US National Institute for Occupational Safety and Health (NIOSH-TR-HHE-75-30-266, PB 273711).

103 GUSEINOV, V.G. (1985) [Toxicological hygienic characteristics of isopropyl alcohol.] *Gig. Tr. Prof. Zabol.,* (7): 60-62 (in Russian).

104 HABU, T., FLATH, R.A., MON, T.R., & MORTON, J.F. (1985) Volatile components of Rooibos tea (*Asphalathus linearis*). *J. agric. food Chem.,* **33**: 249-254.

105 HADDOCK, N.F. & WILKIN J.K. (1982) Cutaneous reactions to lower aliphatic alcohols before and during disulfiram therapy. *Arch. Dermatol.,* **118**: 157-159.

106 HALLIDAY, M.M. & CARTER, K.B. (1978) A chemical adsorption system for the sampling of gaseous organic pollutants in operating theatre atmospheres. *Br. J. Anaesth.,* **50**: 1013-1018.

107 HANSSEN, H.-P., SPRECHER, E., & KLINGENBERG, A. (1984) Accumulation of volatile flavour compounds in liquid cultures of *Kluyveromyces lactis* strains. *Z. Naturforsch.,* **39c**: 1030-1033.

108 HAWLEY, P.C. & FALKO, J.M. (1982) "Pseudo" renal failure after isopropyl alcohol intoxication. *South. med. J.,* **75**: 630-631.

109 HELLMAN, T.M. & SMALL, F.H. (1974) Characterization of the odor properties of 101 petrochemicals using sensory methods. *J. Air Pollut. Control Assoc.*, **24**: 979-982.

110 HERMENS, J. CANTON, H., JANSSEN, P., & DE JONG, R. (1984) Quantitative structure-activity relationships and toxicity studies of mixtures of chemicals with anaesthetic potency: acute lethal and sublethal toxicity to *Daphnia magna*. *Aquat. Toxicol.*, **5**: 143-154.

111 HERMENS, J., BROEKHUYZEN, E., CANTON, H., & WEGMAN, R. (1985) Quantitative structure-activity relationships and mixture toxicity studies of mixtures of alcohols and chlorohydrocarbons: effects on growth of *Daphnia magna*. *Aquat. Toxicol.*, **6**: 209-217.

112 HO, Y.H., SCHWARZE, I., & SOEHRING, K. (1970) [The influence of low aliphatic alcohols on the chloral hydrate metabolism in rat liver sections.] *Arzneim.-Forsch.*, **20**: 1507-1509 (in German).

113 HODGE, H.C. & STERNER, J.H. (1943) *Am. Ind. Hyg. Assoc. J.*, **10**: 93.

114 HOIGNE, J. & BADER, H. (1983) Rate constants of reactions of ozone with organic and inorganic compounds in water. I. Non-dissociating organic compounds. *Water Res.*, **17**: 173-183.

115 HORWITZ, W., ed. (1975) *Official methods of analysis of the Association of Official Analytical Chemists*, 12th ed., Washington DC, Association of Official Analytical Chemists, pp. 328, 337-338, 343, 656-658.

116 HORWOOD, J.F., LLOYD, G.T., & STARK, W. (1981) Some flavour components of feta cheese. *Aust. J. dairy Technol.*, **36**: 34-37.

117 HOU, C.T., PATEL, R.N., LASKIN, A.I., MARCZAK, I., & BARNABE, N. (1981) Microbial oxidation of gaseous hydrocarbons: production of alcohols and methyl ketones from their corresponding *n*- alkanes by methylotrophic bacteria. *Can. J. Microbiol.*, **27**: 107-115.

118 HOVIOUS, J.C., CONWAY, R.A., & GANZE, C.W. (1973) Anaerobic lagoon pretreatment of petrochemical wastes. *J. Water Pollut. Control Fed.*, **45**: 71-84.

119 HUEPER, W.C. (1966) Occupational and environmental cancers of the respiratory system. Recent results. *Cancer Res.*, **3**: 105-107.

120 IARC (1977) *Some fumigants, the herbicides 2,4-D and 2,4,5-T, chlorinated dibenzodioxins and miscellaneous industrial chemicals*, Lyons, International Agency for Research on Cancer, pp. 223-243 (Monographs on the Evaluation of the Carcinogenic Risk of Chemicals to Man, 15).

121 IDOTA, S. (1985) [Studies on isopropanol metabolism and poisoning.] *J. Nihon Univ. Med. Assoc.*, **44**: 39-47 (in Japanese).

122 IRPTC (1987) *Data profile on 2-propanol*, Geneva, Switzerland, International Register of Potentially Toxic Chemicals, United Nations Environment Programme.

123 JARKE, F.H., DRAVNIEKS, A., & GORDON, S.M. (1981) Organic contaminants in indoor air and their relation to outdoor contaminants. *ASHRAE Trans.*, **87**: 153-166.

124 JENSEN, O. (1981) Contact allergy to propylene oxide and isopropyl alcohol in a skin disinfectant swab. *Contact Dermat.*, **7**: 148-150.

125 JONES, C.J. & MCGUGAN, P.J. (1977/1978) An investigation of the evaporation of some volatile solvents from domestic waste. *J. hazard. Mater.*, **2**: 235-251.

126 JONSSON, A., PERSSON, K.A. & GRIGORIADIS, V. (1985) Measurements of some low molecular-weight oxygenated, aromatic, and chlorinated hydrocarbons in ambient air and in vehicle emissions. *Environ. Int.*, **11**: 383-392.

127 JUHNKE, I. & LUDEMANN, D. (1978) [Results of examination of 200 chemical compounds for acute toxicity towards fish by means of the golden orfe test.] *Z. Wasser-Abwasser Forsch.*, **11**: 161-164 (in German).

128 JUNCOS, L. & TAGUCHI, J.T. (1968) Isopropyl alcohol intoxication. Report of a case associated with myopathy, renal failure, and hemolytic anemia. *J. Am. Med. Assoc.*, **204**: 186-188.

129 KAMIL, I.A., SMITH, J.N., & WILLIAMS, R.T. (1953) The metabolism of aliphatic alcohols. The glucuronic acid conjugation of acyclic aliphatic alcohols. *Biochem. J.*, **53**: 129-136.

130 KANE, L.E., DOMBROSKE, R., & ALARIE, Y. (1980) Evaluation of sensory irritation from some common industrial solvents. *Am. Ind. Hyg. Assoc. J.*, **41**: 451-455.

131 KELNER, M. & BAILEY, D.N. (1983) Isopropanol ingestion: interpretation of blood concentrations and clinical findings. *J. Toxicol.-clin. Toxicol.*, **20**: 497-507.

132 KEMAL, H. (1927) [Contribution to investigations into the fate of isopropyl alcohol in the human body.] *Biochem. Z.*, **187**: 461-466 (in German).

133 KHAN, J.S., WILSON, M.C., & TAYLOR, T.V. (1979) A case of dettol addiction. *Br. med. J.*, **1**: 791-792.

References

134 KIMURA, E.T., EBERT, D.M., & DODGE, P.W. (1971) Acute toxicity and limits of solvent residue for sixteen organic solvents. *Toxicol. appl. Pharmacol.*, **19**: 699-703.

135 KING, L.H., BRADLEY, K.P., & SHIRES, D.L. (1970) Hemodialysis for isopropyl alcohol poisoning. *J. Am. Med. Assoc.*, **211**: 1855.

136 KINLIN, T.E., MURALIDHARA, R., PITTET, A.O., SANDERSON, A., & WALRADT, J.P. (1972) Volatile components of roasted filberts. *J. agric. food Chem.*, **20**: 1021-1028.

137 KIRK, R.E. & OTHMER, D.F., ed. (1978-1984) *Encyclopedia of chemical technology*, 3rd ed., New York, Wiley Interscience.

138 KLECKA, G.M. & LANDI, L.P. (1985) Evaluation of the OECD activated sludge, respiration inhibition test. *Chemosphere*, **14**: 1239-1251.

139 KNUTH, M.L. & HOGLUND, M.D. (1984) Quantitative analysis of 68 polar compounds from ten chemical classes by direct aqueous injection gas chromatography. *J. Chromatogr.*, **285**: 153-160.

140 KOMINSKY, J., LOVE, J., & ANDERSON, K. (1982) *Health hazard Evaluation*, Tweddle Litho Company, Cincinnati, Ohio, US National Institute for Occupational Safety and Health (HETA 81-117-1087, PB 83-202390).

141 KONEMANN, H. (1981) Quantitative structure-activity relationships in fish toxicity studies. *Toxicology*, **19**: 209-221.

142 KONIG, H. & HERMES, M. (1981) [Separation, identification and estimation of propellant gases and solvents in aerosol products by gas chromatography.] *Chromatographia*, **14**: 351-354 (in German).

143 KRAMER, V.C., SCHNELL, D.J., & NICKERSON, K.W. (1983) Relative toxicity of organic solvents to *Aedes aegypti* larvae. *J. Invertebr. Pathol.*, **42**: 285-287.

144 KRING, E.V., ANSUL, G.R., HENRY, T.J., MORELLO, J.A., DIXON, S.W., VASTA, J.F., & HEMINGWAY, R.E. (1984) Evaluation of the standard NIOSH type charcoal tube sampling method for organic vapors in air. *Am. Ind. Hyg. Assoc. J.*, **45**: 250-259.

145 KRULL, I.S., SWARTZ, M., & DRISCOLL, J.N. (1984) Derivatizations for improved detection of alcohols by gas chromatography and photoionization detection. *Anal. Lett.*, **17**(A20): 2369-2384.

146 KUMAI, M., KOIZUMI, A., SAITO, K., SAKURAI, H., INOUE, T., TAKEUCHI, Y., HARA, I., OGATA, M., MATSUSHITA, T., & IKEDA, M. (1983) A nationwide survey on organic solvent components in various solvent products. Part 2. Heterogeneous products such as paints, inks, and adhesives. *Ind. Health*, **21**: 185-197.

147 KUMKE, G.W., HALL, J.F., & OEBEN, R.W. (1968) Conversion to activated sludge at Union Carbide's institute plant. *J. Water Pollut. Control Fed.*, **40**: 1408-1422.

148 KURPPA, K. & HUSMAN, K. (1982) Car painters' exposure to a mixture of organic solvents. Serum activities of liver enzymes. *Scand. J. Work environ. Health*, **8**: 137-140.

149 LACOUTURE, P.G., WASON, S., ABRAMS, A., & LOVEJOY, F.H. (1983) Acute isopropyl alcohol intoxication. Diagnosis and management. *Am. J. Med.*, **75**: 680-686.

150 LAHAM, S., POTVIN, M., & SCHRADER, K. (1979) Microméthode de dosage simultané de l'alcool isopropylique et de son métabolite l'acétone. *Chémosphere*, **2**: 79-87.

151 LAHAM, S., POTVIN, M., SCHRADER, K., & MARINO, I. (1980) Studies on inhalation toxicity of 2-propanol. *Drug Chem. Toxicol.*, **3**: 343-360.

152 LANGVARDT, P.W. & MELCHER, R. (1979) Simultaneous determination of polar and non-polar solvents in air using a two-phase desorption from charcoal. *Am. Ind. Hyg. Assoc. J.*, **40**: 1006-1012.

153 LAREGINA, J., BOZZELLI, J.W., HARKOV, R., & GIANTI, S. (1986) Volatile organic compounds at hazardous waste sites and a sanitary landfill in New Jersey. An up-to-date review of the present situation. *Environ. Progr.*, **5**: 18-27.

154 LEASURE, C.S., FLEISCHER, M.E., ANDERSON, G.K., & EICEMAN, G.A. (1986) Photoionization in air with ion mobility spectrometry using a hydrogen discharge lamp. *Anal. Chem.*, **58**: 2142-2147.

155 LEFFINGWELL, S.S., WAXWEILER, R., ALEXANDER, V., LUDWIG, H.R. & HALPERIN, W. (1983) Case-control study of gliomas of the brain among workers employed by a Texas City, Texas chemical plant. *Neuroepidemiology*, **2**: 179-195.

156 LEGENDRE, M.G. & DUPUY, H.P. (1981) *Flavor volatiles as measured by rapid instrumental techniques*, American Chemical Society, pp. 41-49 (ACS Symposium Series No. 147).

157 LEHMAN, A.J. & CHASE, H.F. (1944) The acute and chronic toxicity of isopropyl alcohol. *J. Lab. clin. Med.*, **29**: 561-567.

158 LEHMAN, A.J., SCHWERMA, H., & RICKARDS, E. (1944) Isopropyl alcohol: rate of disappearance from the blood stream of dogs after intravenous and oral administration. *J. Pharmacol. exp. Ther.*, **82**: 196-201.

159 LEHMAN, A.J., SCHWERMA, H., & RICKARDS, E. (1945) Acquired tolerance in dogs, rate of disappearance from the blood stream in various species, and effects on successive generation of rats. *J. Pharmacol. exp. Ther.*, **85**: 61-69.

160 LEWIN, G.A., OPPENHEIMER, P.R., & WINGERT, W.A. (1977) Coma from alcohol sponging. *J.A.C.E.P.*, **6**: 165-167.

161 LEWIS, G.D., LAUFMAN, A.K., MCANALLY, B.H., & GARRIOTT, J.C. (1984) Metabolism of acetone to isopropyl alcohol in rats and humans. *J. forensic Sci.*, **29**: 541-549.

162 LINDSTROM, T.D. & ANDERS, M.W. (1978) Effect of agents known to alter carbon tetrachloride hepatotoxicity and cytochrome P-450 levels on carbon tetrachloride-stimulated lipid peroxidation and ethane expiration in the intact rat. *Biochem. Pharmacol.*, **27**: 563-567.

163 LITOVITZ, T. (1986) The alcohols: ethanol, methanol, iso-propanol, ethylene glycol. *Pediatr. Clin. N. Am.*, **33**: 311-323.

164 LLOYD, A.C., DARNALL, K.R. WINER, A.M., & PITTS, J.N. (1976) Relative rate constants for the reactions of OH radicals with isopropyl alcohol, diethyl and di-n-propyl ether at $305 \pm 20\,°K$. *Chem. Phys. Lett.*, **42**: 205-209.

165 LORR, N.A., MILLER, K.W., CHUNG, H.R., & YANG, C.S. (1984) Potentiation of the hepatotoxicity of N-nitrosodimethylamine by fasting, diabetes, acetone, and isopropanol. *Toxicol. appl. Pharmacol.*, **73**: 423-431.

166 LOVEGREN, N.V., VINNETT, C.H., & ANGELO, A.J.S. (1982) Gas chromatographic profile of good quality raw peanuts. *Peanut Sci.*, **9**: 93-96,

167 LUDWIG, E. & HAUSEN, B.M. (1977) Sensitivity to isopropyl alcohol. *Contact Dermat.*, **3**: 240-244.

168 LUNDBERG, I. & HAKANSSON, M. (1985) Normal serum activities of liver enzymes in Swedish paint industry workers with heavy exposure to organic solvents. *Br. J. ind. Med.*, **42**: 596-600.

169 LYON, R.C., MCCOMB, J.A., SCHREURS, J., & GOLDSTEIN, D.B. (1981) A relationship between alcohol intoxication and the disordering of brain membranes by a series of short-chain alcohols. *J. Pharmacol. exp. Ther.*, **218**: 669-675.

170 MCCORD, W.M., SWITZER, P.K., & BRILL, H.H. (1948) Isopropyl alcohol intoxication. *South med. J.*, **41**: 639-642.

171 MCCREERY, M.J. & HUNT, W.A. (1978) Physico-chemical correlates of alcohol intoxication. *Neuropharmacology*, **17**: 451-461.

172 MCFADDEN, S.W. & HADDOW, J.E. (1969) Coma produced by topical application of isopropanol. *Pediatrics*, **43**: 622-623.

173 MACHYULITE, N.I. (1978) [Hygienic characterization of conditions of work in production of levomycetin.] *Gig. Tr. Prof. Zabol.*, **12**: 8-12 (in Russian).

174 MCINNES, A. (1973) Skin reaction to isopropyl alcohol. *Br. med. J.*, **1**: 357.

175 MACK, K. (1973) The problem of waste water purification in the chemical pharmaceutical industry. *Prog. Water Technol.*, **3**: 239-249.

176 MACK, R.B. (1985) Pervasive procrustianism-isopropyl alcohol intoxication. *N.C. med. J.*, **46**: 101-102.

177 MAIZLISH, N.A., LANGOLF, G.D., WHITEHEAD, L.W., FINE, L.J., ALBERS, J.W., GOLDBERG, J. & SMITH, P. (1985) Behavioural evaluation of workers exposed to mixtures of organic solvents. *Br. J. ind. Med.*, **42**: 579-590.

178 MALILA, A. (1978) Intoxicating effects of three aliphatic alcohols and barbital on two rat strains genetically selected for their ethanol intake. *Pharmacol. Biochem. Behav.*, **8**: 197-201.

179 MARKEL, H. (1982) *Health hazard evaluation, Federal Correctional Institution*, Cincinnati, Ohio, US National Institute for Occupational Safety and Health (HETA 80-119-1066, PB 83-199398).

180 MARTIN, M. & HAERDI, W. (1982) Determination de composes volatils toxiques dans le sang et dans l'urine par chromatographie en phase gazeuse, methode de l'espace de tete (head-space). *Trav. Chim. aliment. Hyg.*, **73**: 212-217.

181 MARTINEZ, T.T., JAEGER, R.W., DECASTRO, F.J., THOMPSON, M.W., & HAMILTON, M.F. (1986) A comparison of the absorption and metabolism of isopropyl alcohol by oral, dermal, and inhalation routes. *Vet. human Toxicol.*, **28**: 233-236.

182 MARZULLI, F.N. & RUGGLES, D.I. (1973) Rabbit eye irritation test: collaborative study. *J. Assoc. Off. Anal. Chem.*, **56**: 905-914.

183 MATSUI, F., LOVERING, E.G., WATSON, J.R., BLACK, D.B., & SEARS, R.W. (1984) Gas chromatographic method for solvent residues in drug raw materials. *J. pharm. Sci.*, **73**: 1664-1666.

184 MATTSON, V.R., ARTHUR, J.W., & WALBRIDGE, C.T. (1976) *Acute toxicity of selected organic compounds to fathead minnows*, Duluth, Minnesota, US Environmental Protection Agency, Environmental Research Laboratory (EPA 600/3-76-097; PB 262897).

185 MAY, J. (1966) [Odour thresholds of solvents for the judgement of solvent odour in air.] *Staub Reinhalt. Luft*, **26**: 385-389 (in German).

186 MECIKALSKI, M.B. & DEPNER, T.A. (1982) Peritoneal dialysis for isopropanol poisoning. *West. J. Med.*, **137**: 322-324.

187 MENDELSON, J., WEXLER, D., LEIDERMAN, P.H., & SOLOMON, P. (1957) A study of addiction to nonethyl alcohols and other poisonous compounds. *Quart. J. Stud. Alcohol*, **18**: 561-580.

188 MORGAN, R.L., SORENSON, S.S., & CASTLES, T.R. (1987) Prediction of ocular irritation by corneal pachymetry. *Food chem. Toxicol.*, **25**: 609-613.

189 MOSHONAS, M.G. & SHAW, P.E. (1972) Analysis of flavor constituents from lemon and lime essence. *J. agric. food Chem.*, **20**: 1029-1030.

190 MUNCH, J.C. (1972) Aliphatic alcohols and alkyl esters: narcotic and lethal potencies to tadpoles and to rabbits. *Ind. Med.*, **41**: 31-33.

191 NATOWICZ, M., DONAHUE, J., GORMAN, L., KANE, M., MCKISSICK, J. & SHAW, L. (1985) Pharmacokinetic analysis of a case of isopropanol intoxication. *Clin. Med.*, **31**: 326-328.

192 NELSON, K.W., EGE, J.F., ROSS, M., WOODMAN, L.E., & SILVERMAN, L. (1943) Sensory response to certain industrial solvent vapors. *J. ind. Hyg. Toxicol.*, **25**: 282-285.

193 NELSON, B.K., BRIGHTWELL, W.S., MACKENZIE-TAYLOR, D.R., KHAN, A., BURG, J.R., WEIGEL, W.W., & GOAD, P.T. (1988) Teratogenicity of *n*-propanol and isopropanol administered at high inhalation concentrations to rats. *Food Chem. Toxicol.*, **26**: 247-254.

194 NIXON, G.A., TYSON, C.A., & WERTZ, W.C. (1975) Interspecies comparisons of skin irritancy. *Toxicol. appl. Pharmacol.*, **31**: 481-490.

195 NORDMANN, R., RIBIERE, C., ROUACH, H., BEAUGE, F., GIUDICELLI, Y., & NORDMANN, J. (1973) Metabolic pathways involved in the oxidation of isopropanol into acetone by the intact rat. *Life Sci.*, **13**: 919-932.

196 OELERT, H.H. & FLORIAN, T. (1972) [Recording and valuation of the inconvenience caused by odours from diesel exhaust.] *Staub Reinhalt. Luft*, **32**: 400-407 (in German).

197 OHASHI, Y., NAKAI, Y., IKEOKA, H., KOSHIMO, H., ESAKI, Y., HORIGUCHI, S., TERAMOTO, K., & NAKASEKO, H. (1987a) Recovery process of tracheal mucosa of guinea-pigs exposed to isopropyl alcohol. *Arch. Toxicol.*, **61**: 12-20.

198 OHASHI, Y., NAKAI, Y., IKEOKA, H., KOSHIMO, H., ESAKI, Y., HORIGUCHI, S., TERAMOTO, K., & NAKASEKO, H. (1987b) Acute effects of isopropyl alcohol exposure on the middle ear mucosa. *J. appl. Toxicol.*, **7**: 205-211.

199 OLSON, B.A. (1982) Effects of organic solvents on behavioural performance of workers in the paint industry. *Neurobehav. Toxicol. Teratol.*, **4**: 703-708.

200 OVEREND, R. & PARASKEVOPOULOS, G. (1978) Rates of OH radical reactions. IV. Reactions with methanol, ethanol, 1-propanol, and 2-propanol at 296 °K. *J. phys. Chem.*, **82**: 1329-1333.

201 PALO, V. & ILKOVA, H. (1970) Direct gas chromatographic estimation of lower alcohols, acetaldehyde, acetone and diacetyl in milk products. *J. Chromatogr.*, **53**: 363-367.

202 PARKER, W.A. (1982-1983) Alcohol-containing pharmaceuticals. *Am. J. drug alcohol Abuse*, **9**: 195-209.

203 PITTER, P. (1976) Determination of biological degradability of organic substances. *Water Res.*, **10**: 231-235.

204 POHL, J. (1922) [Investigations into the fate of methyl and isopropyl alcohol.] *Biochem. Z.*, **127**: 66-71 (in German).

205 POSO, H. & POSO, A.R. (1980) Inhibition by aliphatic alcohols of the stimulated activity of ornithine decarboxylase and tyrosine aminotransferase occurring in regenerating rat liver. *Biochem. Pharmacol.*, **29**: 2799-2803.

206 POWIS, G. (1975) Effect of a single oral dose of methanol, ethanol and propan-2-ol on the hepatic microsomal metabolism of foreign compounds in the rat. *Biochem. J.*, **148**: 269-277.

207 POWIS, G. & GRANT, L. (1976) The effect of inhibitors of alcohol metabolism upon the changes in the hepatic microsomal metabolism of foreign compounds produced by the acute administration of some alcohols to the rat. *Biochem. Pharmacol.*, **25**: 2197-2201.

208 PRICE, K.S., WAGGY, G.T., & CONWAY, R.A. (1974) Brine shrimp bioassay and seawater BOD of petrochemicals. *J. Water Pollut. Control Fed.*, **46**: 63-77.

209 RAICHLE, M.E., EICHLING, J.O., STRAATMANN, M.G., WELCH, M.J., LARSON, K.B., & TER-POGOSSIAN, M.M. (1976) Blood-brain barrier permeability of ^{11}C-labeled alcohols and ^{15}U-labeled water. *Am. J. Physiol.*, **230**: 543-552.

210 RAILE, A., HAMMAN, K.P., SCHEINER, O., SCHULTZ, T., ERDEI, A., & DIERICH, M.P. (1982) Differential effect of low molecular weight alcohols on the Con A stimulation of mouse spleen cells. *Immunol. Lett.*, **4**: 305-309.

211 RAMSEY, J.D. & FLANAGAN, R.J. (1982) Detection and identification of volatile organic compounds in blood by headspace gas chromatograpy as an aid to the diagnosis of solvent abuse. *J. Chromatogr.*, **240**: 423-444.

212 REINDERS, M.E. (1980) *Handbook of emission factors. Part I. Non-industrial sources*, The Hague, Netherlands, Ministry of Health and Environmental Protection.

213 REINHARDT, C.A., PELLI, D.A., & ZBINDEN, G. (1985) Interpretation of cell toxicity data for the estimation of potential irritation. *Food chem. Toxicol.*, **23**: 247-252.

214 REQUENA, J., VELAZ, M.E., GUERRERO, J.R., & MEDINA, J.D. (1985) Isomers of long-chain alkane derivatives and nervous impulse blockage. *J. Membr. Biol.*, **84**: 229-238.

215 REYNOLDS, E.S., MOSLEN, M.T., & TREINEN, R.J. (1982) Isopropanol enhancement of carbon tetrachloride metabolism *in vivo*. *Life Sci.*, **31**: 661-669.

216 REYNOLDS, T. (1977) An anomalous effect of isopropanol on lettuce germination. *Plant Sci. Lett.*, **15**: 25-28.

217 RICHARDSON, D.R., CARAVATI, C.M., PEYTON, E., & WEARY, P.E. (1969) Allergic contact dermatitis to "alcohol" swabs. *Cutis*, **5**: 1115-1118.

218 RIETBROCK, N. & ABSHAGEN, U. (1971) [Pharmacokinetics and metabolism of aliphatic alcohols.] *Arzneim.-Forsch.*, **21**: 1309-1319 (in German).

219 RISTOW, S.S., STARKEY, J.R., & HASS, G.M. (1982) Inhibition of natural killer cell activity *in vitro* by alcohols. *Biochem. Biophys. Res. Commun.*, **105**: 1315-1321.

220 ROSANSKY, S.J. (1982) Isopropyl alcohol poisoning treated with haemodialysis: kinetics of isopropyl alcohol and acetone removal. *J. Toxicol.-clin. Toxicol.*, **19**: 265-271.

221 ROSS, D.H. (1976) Selective action of alcohols on cerebral calcium levels. *Ann. N.Y. Acad. Sci.*, **273**: 280-294.

222 SABLJIC, A. & PROTIC-SABLIC, M. (1983) Quantitative structure-activity study on the mechanism of inhibition of microsomal *p*-hydroxylation of aniline by alcohols. *Mol. Pharmacol.*, **23**: 213-218.

223 SANTODONATO, J. (1985) *Monograph on human exposure to chemicals in the workplace: isopropyl alcohol*, Syracuse, New York, Center for Chemical Hazard Assessment, Syracuse Research Corporation (SRC-TR-84-1043, PB 86-143401).

224 SAVOLAINEN, H., PEKARI, K., & HELOJOKI, H. (1979) Neurochemical and behavioural effects of extended exposure to isopropanol vapour with simultaneous ethanol intake. *Chem.-biol. Interact.*, **28**: 237-248.

225 SAWHNEY, B.L. & KOZLOSKI, R.P. (1984) Organic pollutants in leachates from landfill sites. *J. environ. Qual.*, **13**: 349-352.

226 SCHICK, J.B. & MILSTEIN, J.M. (1981) Burn hazard of isopropyl alcohol in the neonate. *Pediatrics*, **68**: 587-588.

227 SEILER, H., BLAIM, H., & BUSSE, M. (1984) [Antibacterial effects on predominant taxa in the activated sludge system of a chemical combine.] *Z. Wasser-Abwasser Forsch.*, **17**: 127-133 (in German).

228 SENZ, E.H. & GOLDFARB, D.L. (1958) Coma in a child following use of isopropyl alcohol in sponging. *J. Pediatr.*, **53**: 322-323.

229 SHAW, G.J., ALLEN, J.M., & VISSER, F.R. (1985) Volatile flavor components of Babaco fruit (*Carica pentagona*,Heilborn). *J. agric. food Chem.*, **33**: 795-797.

230 SHEHAB, A.S. (1980) Comparative cytological studies of the effect of some aliphatic alcohols and the fatty alcohols from *Euphorbia granulata* and *Pulicaria crispa* on mitosis of *Allium cepa*. *Cytologia*, **45**: 507-513.

231 SHOFSTAHL, J.H. & HARDY, J.K. (1986) Determination of C_1-C_4 alcohols in gasoline using multiple ion detection. *Anal. Chem.*, **58**: 2412-2414.

232 SIEBERT, H., SIEBERT, G., & BOHN, G. (1972) [Animal experimental investigations into the metabolism of propan-2-ol.] *Dtsch. Apoth.-ZTG.*, **112**: 1040-1041 (in German).

233 SINGH, K.V. & AGRAWAL, S.C. (1981) Growth responses of keratinophilic fungi to some volatile substances. *Mykosen*, **24**: 630-634.

234 SIPES, I.G., STRIPP, B., KRISHNA, G., MALING, H., & GILLETTE, J.R. (1973) Enhanced hepatic microsomal activity by pretreatment of rats with acetone or isopropanol. *Proc. Soc. Exp. Biol. Med.*, **142**: 237-240.

235 SMEA (1982) [Problems in industrial toxicology.] (in Russian).

236 SMITH, N.B. (1984) Determination of volatile alcohols and acetone in serum by non-polar capillary gas chromatography after direct sample injection. *Clin. Chem.*, **30**: 1672-1674.

237 SMITH, P. & BROWN, N.L. (1969) Determination of isopropyl alcohol in solid fish protein concentrate by gas-liquid chromatography. *J. agric. food Chem.*, **17**: 34-37.

238 SMITH, R.P. (1959) Poisoning with Old Spice shaving lotion. A case report. *Bull. Suppl. Mat. clin. Toxicol. comm. Prod.*, **2**(11): 12.

239 SMYTH, H.F. & CARPENTER, C.P. (1948) Further experience with the range finding test in the industrial toxicology laboratory. *J. ind. Hyg. Toxicol.*, **30**: 63-70.

240 STEELE, R.H. & WILHELM, D.L. (1966) The inflammatory reaction in chemical injury. I. Increased vascular permeability and erythema induced by various chemicals. *Br. J. exp. Pathol.*, **47**: 612-623.

241 STENSTROM, S., ENLOE, L., PFENNING, M., & RICHELSON, E. (1986) Acute effects of ethanol and other short-chain alcohols on the guanylate cyclase system of murine neuroblastoma cells (clone N1E-115). *J. Pharmacol. exp. Ther.*, **236**: 458-463.

242 STOFBERG, J. & GRUNDSCHOBER, F. (1984) Consumption ratio and food predominance of flavoring materials-second cumulative series. *Perfumer & Flavorist*, **9**: 53-83.

243 STRANGE, A.W., SCHNEIDER, C.W., & GOLDBORT, R. (1976) Selection of C_3 alcohols by high and low ethanol selecting mouse strains and the effects on open field activity. *Pharmacol. Biochem. Behav.*, **4**: 527-530.

244 SWERDEL, M.R. & COUSINS, R.J. (1984) Changes in rat liver metallothionein and metallothionein mRNA induced by isopropanol. *Proc. Soc. Exp. Biol. Med.*, **175**: 522-529.

245 TAYLOR, C.D., COWART, C.O., & RYAN, N.T. (1985) Isopropanol intoxication: managing the coma. *Hosp. Pract.*, **20**: 173-175.

246 TESTA, B. (1981) Structural and electronic factors influencing the inhibition of aniline hydroxylation by alcohols and their binding to cytochrome P-450. *Chem.-biol. Interact.*, **34**: 287-300.

247 TICHY, M., TRCKA, V. ROTH, Z., & KRIVUCOVA, M. (1985) QSAR analysis and data extrapolation among mammals in a series of aliphatic alcohols. *Environ. Health Perspect.*, **61**: 321-328.

248 TIESS, D. & HAMMER, U. (1985) [On endogenous acetone (propane-2-on) and isopropanol (propane-2-ol) levels in the human body after ketoacidic states.] *Z. gesamte Hyg.*, **31**: 527-529 (in German).

249 TIMMER, R., TER HEIDE, R., DE VALOIS, P.J., & WOBBEN, H.J. (1971) Qualitative analysis of the most volatile neutral components of Reunion geranium oil (*Pelargonium roseum* Bourbon). *J. agric. food Chem.*, **19**: 1066-1068.

250 TOMITA, M. & NISHIMURA, M. (1982) Using saliva to estimate human exposure to organic solvents. *Bull. Tokyo dent. Coll.*, **23**: 175-188.

251 TOOBY, T.E., HURSEY, P.A., & ALABASTER, J.S. (1975) The acute toxicity of 102 pesticides and miscellaneous substances to fish. *Chem. Ind.*, **12**: 523-526.

252 TRAIGER, G.J. & PLAA, G.L. (1972) Relationship of alcohol metabolism to the potentiation of CCl_4 hepatotoxicity induced by aliphatic alcohols. *J. Pharmacol. exp. Ther.*, **183**: 481-488.

253 TRAIGER, G.J. & PLAA, G.L. (1974) Chlorinated hydrocarbon toxicity. Potentiation by isopropyl alcohol and acetone. *Arch. environ. Health*, **28**: 276-278.

254 TU, Y.Y., PENG, R., CHANG, Z.-F., & YANG, C.S. (1983) Induction of a high affinity nitrosamine demethylase in rat liver microsomes by acetone and isopropanol. *Chem.-biol. Interact.*, **44**: 247-260.

255 UENG, T.-H., MOORE, L., ELVES, R.G., & ALVARES, A.P. (1983) Isopropanol enhancement of cytochrome P-450-dependent monooxygenase activities and its effects on carbon tetrachloride intoxication. *Toxicol. appl. Pharmacol.*, **71**: 204-214.

256 URANO, K., OGURA, K., & WADA, H. (1981) Direct analytical method for aliphatic compounds in water by steam carrier gas chromatography. *Water Res.*, **15**: 225-231.

257 US NIOSH (1976) *Criteria for a recommended standard: occupational exposure to isopropyl alcohol*, Cincinnati, Ohio, US National Institute of Occupational Safety and Health, US Department of Health, Education, and Welfare, Public Health Services, Center for Disease Control (DHEW Publication No. (NIOSH)76-142).

258 US NIOSH (1977) *Manual of analytical methods*, 2nd ed., Cincinnati, Ohio, US National Institute for Occupational Safety and Health, US Department of Health, Education, and Welfare, Vol. 2, pp. S185.

259 US NIOSH (1984) Method 1400. In: Eller, P.M., ed. NIOSH *Manual of analytical methods*, 3rd ed., Cincinnati, Ohio, National Institute for Occupational Safety and Health, Vol. 1, pp. 1400-11400-5.

260 VAN RILLAER, W.G. & BEERNAERT, H. (1983) Determination of residual isopropanol and propylene glycol in soft drinks by glass capillary gas chromatography. *Z. Lebensm. Unters. Forsch.*, **177**: 196-199.

References

261 VASILIADES, J., POLLOCK, J., & ROBINSON, C.A. (1978) Pitfalls of the alcohol dehydrogenase procedure for the emergency assay of alcohol: a case study of isopropanol overdose. *Clin. Chem.*, **24**: 383-385.

262 VEITH, G.D. & KOSIAN, P. (1983) Estimating bioconcentration potential from octanol/water partition coefficients. In: Mackay et al., ed. *Physical behaviour of PCBs in the Great Lakes*, Ann Arbor, Michigan, Ann Arbor Science, pp. 269-282.

263 VEITH, G.D., CALL, D.J., & BROOKE, L.T. (1983) Structure-toxicity relationships for the fathead minnow, *Pimephales promelas*: narcotic industrial chemicals. *Can. J. Fish. aquat. Sci.*, **40**: 743-748.

264 VIDELA, L.A., FERNANDEZ, V., & DE MARINIS, A. (1982) Liver peroxidative pressure and glutathione status following acetaldehyde and aliphatic alcohols pretreatment in the rat. *Biochem. Biophys. Res. Commun.*, **104**: 965-970.

265 VILAGELIU ARQUES, L. & GONZALEZ DUARTE, R. (1980) Effect of ethanol and isopropanol on the activity of alcohol dehydrogenase, viability and life-span in *Drosophila melanogaster* and *Drosophila funebris*. *Experientia*, **36**: 828-830.

266 VISUDHIPAN, P. & KAUFMAN, H. (1971) Increased cerebrospinal fluid protein following isopropyl alcohol intoxication. *N.Y. State J. Med.*, **71**: 887-880.

267 VON DER HUDE, W., SCHEUTWINKEL, M., GRAMLICH, U., FISSLER, B., & BUSLER, A. (1987) Genotoxicity of three carbon compounds evaluated in the SCE test *in vitro*. *Environ. Mutagen.*, **9**: 401-410.

268 WAGNER, R. (1974) [Investigations into the degradation behaviour of organic compounds using the respirometric dilution method. I. Monohydric alcohols.] *Vom Wasser*, **42**: 271-305 (in German).

269 WAGNER, R. (1976) [Investigations into the degradation behaviour of organic compounds using the respirometric dilution method. II. The degradation kinetics of the test compounds.] *Vom Wasser*, **47**: 241-265 (in German).

270 WALLGREN, H. (1960) Relative intoxicating effects on rats of ethyl, propyl and butyl alcohols. *Acta pharmacol. toxicol.*, **16**: 217-222.

271 WALLINGFORD, K.M. (1983) *Health hazard evaluation, Xomox Corporation*, Cincinnati, Ohio, US National Institute for Occupational Safety and Health (HETA 83-170-1346, PB 85-163434).

272 WASILEWSKI, C. (1968) Allergic contact dermatitis from isopropyl alcohol. *Arch. Dermatol.*, **98**: 502-504.

273 WATERER, D.R. & PRITCHARD, M.K. (1984) Monitoring of volatiles: a technique for detection of soft rot (*Erwinia carotovora*) in potato tubers. *Can. J. Plant. Pathol.*, **6**: 165-171.

274 WAX, J., ELLIS, F.W., & LEHMAN, A.J. (1949) Absorption and distribution of isopropyl alcohol. *J. Pathol. exp. Ther.*, **97**: 229-237.

275 WEBBER, D. (1984) Basic chemical output returns to growth. Top 50 chemical products. *Chem. eng. News*, **May 7**: 8-10.

276 WEIL, C.S., SMYTH, H.F., & NALE, T.W. (1952) Quest for a suspected industrial carcinogen. *Arch. ind. Hyg. occup. Med.*, **5**: 535-547.

277 WEINTRAUB, Z. & IANCU, T.C. (1982) Isopropyl alcohol burns. *Pediatrics*, **69**: 506.

278 WHITE, G.A., EMMETT, E.A., KOMINSKY, J.R., & SINGAL, M. (1983) *Health hazard evaluation, Inland Division, GMC*, Cincinnati, Ohio, US National Institute for Occupational Safety and Health (HETA 77-011-1338, PB 85-101319).

279 WHITEHEAD, L.W., BALL, G.L., FINE, L.J., & LANGOLF, G.D. (1984) Solvent vapor exposures in booth spray painting and spray glueing, and associated operations. *Am. ind. Hyg. Assoc. J.*, **45**: 767-772.

280 WILKINSON, C. & IGLEWICZ, R. (1982) *Health hazard evaluation, Syntrex Corporation*, Cincinnati, Ohio, US National Institute for Occupational Safety and Health (HETA 81-370-1050, PB 83-198424).

281 WILKINSON, T. & HAMER, G. (1979) The microbial oxidation of mixtures of methanol, phenol, acetone, and isopropanol with reference to effluent purification. *J. chem. Technol. Biotechnol.*, **29**: 56-67.

282 WILLIAMS, T.M., HICKEY, J.L.S., & SHY, C.M. (1982) *Health hazard evaluation, Dittler Brothers, Inc.*, Cincinnati, Ohio, US National Institute for Occupational Safety and Health (HETA 81-173-1051, PB 83-198473).

283 WILLS, J.H., JAMESON, E.M., & COULSTON, F. (1969) Effects on man of daily ingestion of small doses of isopropyl alcohol. *Toxicol. appl. Pharmacol.*, **15**: 560-565.

284 WINEK, C.L. & JANSSEN, J.K. (1982) Blood versus bone marrow isopropanol concentrations in rabbits. *Forensic Sci. Int.*, **20**: 11-20.

285 WOLFF, T. (1978) In vitroinhibition of monooxygenase dependent reactions by organic solvents. *Int. Congr. Ser. Excerpta Med.*, **440**: 196-199.

286 WRIGHT, U. (1979) The hidden carcinogen in the manufacture of isopropyl alcohol. *Dev. Toxicol. environ. Sci.*, **4**: 93-98.

References

287 YASHUDA, Y., CABRAL, A.M., & ANTONIO, A. (1976) Inhibitory action of aliphatic alcohols on smooth muscle contraction. *Pharmacology*, **14**: 473-478.

288 YOUNG, P.J. & PARKER, A. (1983) The identification and possible environmental impact of trace gases and vapours in landfill gas. *Waste Management Res.*, **1**: 213-226.

289 YOUNG, R.H.F., RYCKMAN, D.W., & BUZZELL, J.C. (1968) An improved tool for measuring biodegradability. *J. Water Pollut. Control Fed.*, **40**: R354-R368.

290 ZAHLSEN, K., AARSTAD, K., & NILSEN, O.G. (1985) Inhalation of isopropanol: induction of activating and deactivating enzymes in rat kidney and liver, increased microsomal metabolism of *n*-hexane. *Toxicology*, **34**: 57-66.

291 ZAKHARI, S. (1977) *Isopropanol and ketones in the environment*, Oxford, England, CRC Press.

292 ZINBO, M. (1984) Determination of one-carbon to three-carbon alcohols and water in gasoline/alcohol blends by liquid chromatography. *Anal. Chem.*, **56**: 244-247.

RESUME

1. **Identité, propriétés physiques et chimiques, méthodes d'analyse**

   Le propanol-2 est un liquide incolore, très inflammable dont l'odeur rappelle celle d'un mélange d'éthanol et d'acétone. Il est entièrement miscible à l'eau, à l'éthanol, à l'acétone, au chloroforme et au benzène. Il existe des méthodes d'analyse pour la recherche du propanol-2 dans divers milieux (air, eau, sang, sérum et urine), avec des limites de détection dans l'air, l'eau et le sang respectivement égales à 2×10^{-5} mg/m^3, 0,04 mg/litre et 1 mg/litre. La chromatographie en phase gazeuse (essentiellement avec détection par ionisation de flamme) ainsi que l'électrophorèse sur papier et la spectrométrie de mobilité ionique par photoionisation permettent de doser le propanol-2 dans divers mileux.

2. **Sources d'exposition humaine et environnementale**

   On estime qu'en 1975, la production mondiale de propanol-2 dépassait 1100 kilotonnes, la capacité mondiale de production étant supérieure à 2000 kilotonnes en 1984. Le propanol-2 est couramment produit à partir du propène. Les procédés antérieurs de fabrication qui reposaient sur l'utilisation d'acides forts ou d'acides faibles, et donnaient naissance à des produits intermédiaires et à des sous-produits potentiellement dangereux, sont désormais largement supplantés par le procédé d'hydratation catalytique. On peut également procéder par réduction catalytique de l'acétone.

   Le propanol-2 est un produit du métabolisme de divers microorganismes.

   Il a de nombreuses applications comme solvant et il entre dans la composition de différents produits ménagers et produits de soins personnels, sous forme d'aérosols et d'excipients pour produits pharmaceutiques à usage externe et pour cosmétiques. Le propanol-2 est également utilisé pour la production de l'acétone et autres produits chimiques, comme agent de dégivrage, comme conservateur et il entre dans la composition des concentrés pour le nettoyage des pare-brise et de certains aromatisants alimentaires.

Le propanol-2 peut pénétrer dans l'atmosphère, dans l'eau et dans le sol lors du rejet de déchets et on en a trouvé dans l'air et dans les eaux de lessivage de décharges mal protégées. Présent dans les gaz et eaux résiduaires industriels, on peut l'en éliminer par oxydation biologique ou osmose inverse. Il peut être dissipé dans l'atmosphère lors de l'utilisation de produits de consommation qui en contiennent.

3. Transport et distribution dans l'environnement

C'est principalement lors d'opérations telles que la production, la transformation, le stockage, le transport, l'utilisation et le rejet de déchets que le propanol-2 pénètre dans l'environnement atmosphérique. Il peut être également déchargé dans le sol et l'eau. Il est difficile d'évaluer la part qui revient à chaque compartiment du milieu. Toutefois on estimait en 1976 que plus de 50 % du propanol-2 produit finissait par être libéré dans l'atmosphère.

Le propanol-2 est rapidement éliminé de l'atmosphère par réaction sur les radicaux hydroxyles et entraînement par les précipitations. Ce sont ces dernières qui sont responsables du transport de ce composé de l'atmosphère dans le sol ou l'eau. Une fois dans le sol, il doit y être très mobile et augmente la perméabilité du sol à certains hydrocarbures aromatiques. Le propanol-2 est facilement biodégradable par voie aérobie ou anaérobie.

Comme il est biodégradable et complètement miscible à l'eau, avec un coefficient de partition octanol/eau logarithmique de 0,14 et un facteur de bioconcentration de 0,5, il est peu probable qu'il donne lieu à une bioaccumulation.

4. Niveaux dans l'environnement et exposition humaine

L'exposition de la population en général peut se produire par ingestion accidentelle ou volontaire, par absorption de nourriture contenant du propanol-2 d'origine naturelle, ou sous forme d'aromatisant volatil ou de résidus de solvant, ou encore par inhalation lors de l'utilisation de produits qui en contiennent. On en a trouvé aux concentrations de 0,2 à 325 mg/litre dans des boissons non alcoolisées et aux concentrations de 50 à 3000 mg/kg dans des denrées alimentaires pour la production desquelles on l'avait utilisé comme solvant. L'exposition de la population en général par inhalation de l'air ambiant est faible, du fait de l'élimination et de la dégradation rapides de ce produit. En procédant à des contrôles en divers lieux et, en particulier, dans des sites urbains, on a obtenu des concentrations moyennes pondérées par rapport au temps allant jusqu'à 35 mg/m^3.

Les travailleurs peuvent être exposés au propanol-2 au cours de la production du composé lui-même, lors de la fabrication de l'acétone ou d'autres dérivés et également lorsqu'on utilise ce produit comme solvant. Aux Etats-Unis, une enquête (National Occupational Exposure Survey) effectuée en 1980-83 a montré que plus de 1,8 million de travailleurs pouvaient être exposés. On a mesuré sur les lieux de travail des concentrations atteignant 1350 mg/m^3 avec des moyennes pondérées par rapport au temps allant jusqu'á 500 mg/m^3.

5. Cinétique et métabolisme

Le propanol-2 est rapidement absorbé et se répartit dans tout l'organisme par inhalation et ingestion. A forte dose, l'absorption dans les voies digestives est retardée. Les taux sanguins de propanol-2 (décelables lorsqu'il y a ingestion simultanée d'éthanol) ou de son métabolite, l'acétone, sont corrélés avec l'intensité de l'exposition. Des volontaires qui avaient ingéré une dose de 3,75 mg/kg de propanol-2 (avec 1200 mg d'éthanol/kg) dans du jus d'orange, présentaient une concentration sanguine maximale de propanol-2 libre de $0,8 \pm 0,3$ mg/litre, et de $2,3 \pm 1,4$ mg/litre après incubation en présence d'arylsulfatase, ce qui témoigne d'une sulfatation. Chez les ouvriers exposés à des vapeurs de propanol-2 (8–647 mg/m^3), on a observé des concentrations de 3–270 mg/m^3 dans l'air alvéolaire, mais dans ce cas, c'est de l'acétone et non du propanol-2 que l'on a trouvé dans le sang et les urines. Chez des animaux de laboratoire exposés au propanol-2, on a retrouvé celui-ci non seulement dans le sang mais également dans le liquide céphalo-rachidien, dans le foie, les reins et le cerveau. Le propanol-2 traverse la barrière hémo-méningée deux fois plus facilement que l'éthanol. Le propanol-2 est excrété en partie tel quel et en partie sous forme d'acétone, essentiellement au niveau des poumons mais également dans la salive et le suc gastrique. Il peut y avoir réabsorption après excrétion par ces deux dernières voies. La métabolisation en acétone en présence d'alcool-déshydrogénase (ADH) hépatique est assez lente, du fait que l'ADH a une moindre affinité pour le propanol-2 que pour l'éthanol. *In vitro*, l'activité de l'ADH humaine vis-à-vis du propanol-2 correspond à 9-10 % de l'activité de cette enzyme lorsque le substrat est de l'éthanol. Les oxydases microsomiques du foie de rat sont également capables d'oxyder le propanol-2 *in vitro*. Chez l'homme, l'acétone est excrétée telle quelle, essentiellement au niveau des poumons et en quantité minime au niveau des reins. Plus l'exposition au propanol-2 se prolonge, plus la concentration d'acétone dans l'air alvéolaire, dans le sang et dans les urines est élevée. Le propanol-2 et l'acétone sont éliminés de l'organisme selon une cinétique du premier ordre et leur demi-vie chez l'homme est de 2,5–6,4 heures et 22 heures, respectivement.

6. Effets sur les êtres vivants dans leur milieu naturel

Le propanol-2 est peu toxique pour la faune et la flore aquatiques, les insectes et les plantes. Son seuil d'inhibition de la multiplication cellulaire, mesuré chez une espèce sensible de protozoaire, varie de 104 à 4930 mg/litre selon les conditions expérimentales. Si l'on s'élève dans l'arbre phylogénétique, on constate que diverses espèces de crustacés, notamment *Daphnia magna*, présentent des CE_{50} allant de 2285 à 9714 mg/litre. Pour des poissons d'eau douce, on a obtenu des CL_{50} à 96 heures allant de 4200 à 11 130 mg/litre. Chez la drosophile, les CL_{50} vont de 10 200 à 13 340 mg/litre de milieu nutritif. Pour le troisième stade larvaire du moustique *Aedes aegypti*, on a obtenu, lors d'une épreuve statique de 4 heures, des valeurs de la CL_{50} allant de 25 à 120 mg/litre.

L'exposition de végétaux à du propanol-2 à des concentrations comprises entre 2100 mg/litre et plus de 36 000 mg/litre, a provoqué toute une gamme d'effets allant de l'absence totale d'anomalies à une inhibition complète de la germination.

Résumé

7. Effets sur les animaux d'expérience et les systèmes d'épreuves *in vitro*

A en juger d'après la mortalité qu'il provoque, le propanol-2 présente une faible toxicité aiguë pour les mammifères, que l'exposition ait lieu par voie orale, percutanée ou respiratoire. Chez plusieurs espèces animales on a obtenu, après administration par voie orale, des valeurs de la DL_{50} allant de 4475 à 7990 mg par kg de poids corporel; la CL_{50} pour une inhalation de 8 heures allait de 46 000 à 56 000 mg/m^3 d'air chez le rat. A ces doses mortelles, les rats présentaient une forte irritation des muqueuses et une grave dépression du système nerveux central. La mort est survenue par arrêt cardiaque ou respiratoire. Entre autres lésions histopathologiques, on notait une congestion et un oedème du poumon ainsi qu' une dégénérescence des hépatocytes.

Administré en dose unique par voie orale à des rats à raison de 3000 ou 6000 mg par kg de poids corporel, le propanol-2 a provoqué une accumulation réversible de triglycérides dans le foie. On a également observé chez ces rats une induction des enzymes microsomiques à la dose de 390 mg/kg.

Non dilué, le propanol-2 n'est pas irritant en applications de 4 heures sur la peau, intacte ou abrasée, de lapins tondus. Toutefois, en instillations oculaires de 0,1 ml, le propanol-2 non dilué a provoqué une irritation chez le lapin. De fortes concentrations de vapeurs de propanol-2 ont provoqué une irritation respiratoire chez la souris et l'on a noté une réduction de 50 % du rythme respiratoire à des concentrations allant de 12 300 à 43 525 mg/m^3 d'air.

Les études conscrées aux effets sur l'animal d'exposition répétées au propanol-2 sont plutôt limitées. Après inhalation par des rats de 500 mg/m^3 de propanol-2, cinq jours par semaine et quatre heures par jour pendant quatre mois, on a noté une irritation des voies respiratoires, des anomalies haématologiques et des altérations histopathologiques au niveau du foie et de la rate. Un autre groupe expérimental composé de cinq rats de chaque sexe a reçu pendant 27 semaines du propanol-2 dans son eau de boisson. En comparant les animaux qui recevaient environ 600 ou 2300 mg/kg par jour (mâles) et 1000 ou 3900 mg/kg par jour (femelles) de propanol-2 à des témoins non traités, on a constaté un retard de croissance, mais uniquement chez les deux groupes de femelles traitées. Aucun autre effet indésirable n'a été constaté.

Les données disponibles donnent à penser que le propanol-2 produit sur le système nerveux central (SNC) des effets analogues à ceux de l'éthanol. La DE_{50} d'anésthésie par voie orale est de 2280 mg/kg chez le lapin, la DE_{50} par voie intrapéritonéale correspondant à la perte du réflexe de redressement chez la souris est égale à 165 mg/kg et le seuil d'induction de l'ataxie par voie intrapéritonéale est de 1106 mg/kg chez le rat. Ces valeurs sont sont environ deux fois plus faibles que pour l'éthanol. Lors d'une expérience menée à l'air libre, on a constaté que l'inhalation de propanol-2 à la dose de 739 mg/m^3, dix heures par jour, et cinq jours par semaine pendant 15 semaines ne produisait aucun effet indésirable.

Le propanol-2 a été soumis à une étude portant sur deux générations de rats qui ont reçu dans leur eau de boisson des doses quotidiennes de 1290, 1380 ou 1479 mg de ce produit par kg de poids corporel. Les seuls effets indésirables qui ont été notés consistaient dans une réduction passagère du taux de croissance dans la génération F_0. En revanche, d'autres chercheurs ont constaté une augmentation des malformations lors d'une étude tératogènicité, au cours de laquelle on avait administré à des rates gravides, des doses orales quotidiennes de 252 ou 1008 mg de propanol-2 par kg de poids corporel (toxicité maternelle non étudiée). On a également indiqué que ces deux doses, administrées pendant 45 jours dans l'eau de boisson, faisaient passer le cycle oestral à cinq jours (contre quatre chez les témoins). Chez des rates ayant reçu pendant six mois dans leur eau de boisson, des doses quotidiennes de propanol-2 de 1800 mg/kg avant de mettre bas, on a constaté un accroissement de la mortalité embryonnaire totale; divers effets ont également été signalés concernant la survie intra-utérine et postnatale à des doses aussi basses que 0,8 mg/kg, sans qu'on puisse toutefois dégager une tendance précise. Des rates gravides ont été exposées à de l'air contenant du propanol-2 aux concentrations respectives de 9001, 18 327 et 23 210 mg/m^3 (3659, 7450 ou 9435 ppm). Les deux concentrations les plus fortes se sont révélées toxiques pour les mères, la concentration de

9001 mg/m³ ne produisant aucun effet. A toutes les concentrations on a constaté un effet nocif sur le développement.

Une épreuve de recherche des mutations ponctuelles utilisant *S. typhimurium* a donné des résultats négatifs avec du propanol-2 à la dose de 0,18 mg par boîte; la recherche d'échanges entre chromatides soeurs sur fibroblastes de hamster chinois a également été négative. Le propanol-2 a provoqué des anomalies de la mitose dans des cellules médullaires de rat ainsi que des cellules de l'extrémité radiculaire d'oignons *in vitro*. On ne dispose d'aucune autre donnée sur la mutagénicité de ce produit.

Un certain nombre d'études restreintes ont été consacrées au pouvoir cancérogène du propanol-2, au cours desquelles des souris ont été exposées à cette substance par voie percutanée (3 fois par semaine pendant un an), par voie respiratoire (7700 mg/m³, 3 à 7 heures par jour, cinq jours par semaine pendant 5 à 8 mois) et par voie sous-cutanée (20 mg de propanol non dilué par semaine pendant 20 à 40 semaines). Au cours de ces trois études, on a recherché la présence de tumeurs sur la peau, dans les poumons et au point d'injection. Aucun signe d'effets cancérogènes n'a été observé. On ne dispose pas de données épidémiologiques suffisantes pour évaluer la cancérogénicité du propanol-2 chez l'homme. A la lumière des données disponibles, on peut penser que le sulfate de dipropyl-2, un produit intermédiaire de la fabrication du propanol-2 par le procédé aux acides forts et faibles, pourrait être à l'origine de cancers du sinus maxillaire chez l'homme.

8. Effets sur la santé de l'homme

On a signalé plusieurs cas d'intoxication consécutifs à l'ingestion de propanol-2 ou à l'utilisation de lotions à base de ce produit pour rafraîchir des enfants fébriles. Les principaux signes d'intoxication rappellent ceux de l'intoxication alcoolique : nausées, vomissements, douleurs abdominales, gastrite, hypotension et hypothermie. La dépression du SNC par le propanol-2 est deux fois plus intense qu'avec l'éthanol et entraîne l'inconscience puis un coma profond; la mort peut survenir par dépression respiratoire. Parmi les autres effets on peut noter l'hyperglycémie, un taux élevé de protéines dans le liquide céphalorachidien et une atélectasie. Il semblerait que l'absorption percutanée soit négligeable mais on connaît le cas d'un enfant qui a été intoxiqué après avoir été lotionné avec du propanol-2, ce qui donne à penser qu'il ne faut pas négliger l'absorption percutanée, notamment chez les enfants. Aucun effet indésirable n'a été observé chez des volontaires en bonne santé qui avaient bu tous les jours pendant six semaines un sirop contenant du propanol-2 à des doses corrrespondant respectivement à 2,6 et 6,4 mg de propanol-2 par kg de poids corporel. Des volontaires du sexe masculin, exposés 3 à 5 minutes à des vapeurs de propanol-2 correspondant à des concentrations de 490, 980 ou 1970 mg/m^3 d'air, ont estimé qu'ils ressentaient une irritation légère à 980 mg/m^3 et que la situation était "satisfaisante" pendant les 8 heures correspondant à leur propre exposition professionnelle.

Des enfants prématurés ayant subi un contact prolongé avec du propanol-2 ont présenté une irritation cutanée prenant la forme d'érythèmes, voire de brûlures du 2ème et du 3ème degré et de phlyctènes. On a également signalé ça et là des cas de dermatites allergiques de contact.

Il n'existe de peu d'études épidémiologiques consacrées à la mortalité par cancers ou autres maladies provoquées par le propanol-2. Parmi un groupe de 61 travailleurs, employés pendant plus de cinq ans dans un atelier de fabrication de propanol-2 par le procédé à l'acide fort, on a observé sept cas de cancer dont quatre de cancer des sinus maxillaires. Une étude portant sur une cohorte de 779 travailleurs d'un atelier analogue a révélé que l'incidence des cancers du sinus et du larynx, corrigée de l'influence de l'âge et du sexe, était 21 fois plus forte que prévue. La période minimale de latence était de dix ans. Dans une autre étude rétrospective de cohorte portant sur le personnel d'une autre usine où on utilisait le procédé à l'acide fort, on a constitué une cohorte représentant plus de 4000 années-hommes exposés au risque. Les résultats de cette étude ont montré que les taux de mortalité pour toutes causes et les taux de mortalité par cancer n'étaient pas sensiblement plus élevés que les taux prévisibles. Une autre étude rétrospective a été menée dans une usine qui fabriquait du propanol-2 par le procédé à l'acide faible. Cette fois, on comptait plus de 11 000 années-hommes exposés au risque. Dans ce cas, le taux de mortalité pour toutes causes était inférieur aux prévisions et l'on ne constatait pas de surmortalité attribuable aux cancers en général. Toutefois, l'incidence des cancers de la bouche et du pharynx était 4 fois supérieure à la normale. Dans l'ensemble, ces études de cohorte donnent à penser qu'il existe un risque de cancer imputable au procédé à l'acide fort; toutefois lors de deux petites études cas-témoins, on n'a noté aucune association entre l'exposition au propanol-2 et l'incidence des gliomes ou de la leucémie lymphatique.

Certaines études font état d'une potentialisation de la toxicité du tétrachlorure de carbone chez des ouvriers simultanément exposés au propanol-2.

9. Résumé de l'évaluation

L'homme peut être exposé au propanol-2 par inhalation lors de la fabrication, de la transformation ou de l'utilisation de cette substance dans le cadre professionnel ou domestique. En ce qui concerne la population en général, l'exposition à des doses potentiellement mortelles peut se produire par suite d'ingestion accidentelle ou volontaire de cette substance et les enfants peuvent être exposés par application de lotions à base de propanol-2.

Le propanol-2 est vite absorbé et se répartit rapidement dans l'ensemble de l'organisme, en partie sous forme d'acétone. Les données relatives aux effets aigus consécutifs à l'exposition d'êtres humains à des doses excessives sont rares et contrastées. Les principaux effets consistent en gastrite, dépression du système nerveux central, hypothermie, dépression respiratoire et hypotension. Les données de mortalité aiguë obtenues sur des animaux de laboratoire indiquent que le propanol-2 est peu toxique, les valeurs de la DL_{50} par voie orale chez diverses espèces vont de 4475 à 7990 mg/kg, et les valeurs de la CL_{50} par inhalation se situent aux alentours de 50 000 mg/m^3 chez le rat. Chez le lapin, le propanol-2 ne provoque pas d'irritation cutanée, toutefois l'instillation de 0,1 ml de cette substance non diluée dans les yeux a provoqué une irritation.

Chez l'homme, les effets aigus les plus probables d'une exposition de fortes concentrations de propanol-2 par ingestion ou inhalation, consistent en une intoxication de type alcoolique aboutissant à la narcose.

Les études sur l'animal sont insuffisantes pour qu'on puisse évaluer les risques encourus par l'homme à la suite d'expositions répétées au propanol-2. Toutefois les résultats de deux études à court terme chez le rat, au cours desquelles on a fait a) inhaler 500 mg/m^3 de cette substance, 4 heures par jour, 5 heures par semaine pendant 4 mois et b) ingérer le même produit à raison de 600 à 3900 mg/kg dans l'eau de boisson, donnent à penser qu'il serait préférable d'éviter de s'exposer aux fortes concentrations en propanol-2 signalées dans le cadre de certaines activités professionnelles.

En faisant inhaler du propanol-2 à des rattes gravides on a constaté que le seuil d'apparition d'un effet se situait à 18 327 mg/m^3 (7450 ppm), la dose sans effet observable était de 9001 mg/m^3 (3659 ppm), la toxicité maternelle étant prise comme critère. Au cours de la même étude, le seuil d'apparition d'effets s'est situé à 9001 mg/m^3 (3659 ppm) pour les anomalies du développement et aucune dose sans effet observable n'a pu être mise en évidence. Ces concentrations sont plus élevées que celles auxquelles l'homme est susceptible d'être exposé.

Les épreuves de génotoxicité ont donné des résultats négatifs dans le cas du propanol-2, cependant on a observé des anomalies de la mitose dans des cellules médullaires de rats. Ces résultats indiquent que le propanol-2 n'est pas du tout génétoxique mais les données sont trop limitées pour qu'on puisse se prononcer véritablement sur le pouvoir mutagène de cette substance.

Les données existantes sont insuffisantes pour permettre une évaluation de la cancérogénicité du propanol-2 chez l'animal d'expérience. On ne dispose pas de données permettant d'évaluer cette cancérogénicité chez l'homme.

Le propanol-2 ne fait probablement pas courir de risque important à la population dans son ensemble dans les conditions d'exposition qui sont susceptibles de se produire.

Le propanol-2 disparaît rapidement (demi-vie, 5 jours) de l'atmosphère et s'élimine à bref délai de l'eau et du sol par biodégradation aérobie ou anaérobie, en particulier une fois que les microorganismes préalablement ensemencés se sont adaptés. Compte tenu de ses propriétés physiques, le propanol-2 n'a qu'une faible tendance à la bioaccumulation. Il ne présente pas de risque pour la faune et la flore aux concentrations auxquelles il est habituellement présent dans l'environnement.

RESUMEN

1. Identidad, propiedades físicas y químicas, métodos analíticos

   El 2-propanol es un líquido incoloro, sumamente inflamable, con un olor que recuerda al de la mezcla de etanol y acetona. El compuesto es completamente miscible con agua, etanol, acetona, cloroformo y benceno. Se dispone de métodos analíticos para detectar el 2-propanol en diversos medios (aire, agua, sangre, suero y orina) con límites de detección de 2×10^{-5} mg/m^3, 0,04 mg/litro y 1 mg/litro en el aire, el agua y la sangre, respectivamente. Existen métodos de cromatografía de gases (que se sirven principalmente de la detección de ionización de llama) así como métodos de electroforesis en papel y de espectrometría de movilidad iónica inducida por fotoionización para determinar el 2-propanol en los distintos medios.

2. Fuentes de exposición humana y ambiental

   La producción mundial estimada de 2-propanol en 1975 fue superior a 1100 kilotoneladas y la capacidad de producción mundial en 1984 se cifró en más de 2000 kilotoneladas. El 2-propanol se fabrica comúnmente a partir del propeno. Los antiguos procesos basados en ácidos fuertes y débiles, en los que se generaban productos intermedios y desechos potencialmente peligrosos, se han sustituido actualmente en gran medida por el proceso de hidratación catalítica. La reducción catalítica de la acetona es otro proceso posible.

   El 2-propanol se ha identificado como producto metabólico de diversos microorganismos.

   El compuesto tiene amplias aplicaciones como disolvente y se utiliza como componente de productos domésticos y personales, entre ellos vaporizadores de aerosoles, productos farmacéuticos de aplicación tópica y cosméticos. El 2-propanol se utiliza también para producir acetona y otras sustancias químicas, como agente descongelante, como conservante, en concentrados para limpiaparabrisas y como aromatizante volátil en alimentos.

El 2-propanol puede ingresar en la atmósfera, el agua o el suelo por la evacuación de desechos y se ha aislado en el aire y en el líquido que rezuma de basureros y terraplenados. Se encuentra en los gases y las aguas residuales que emiten algunas industrias, y puede extraerse de esas aguas por oxidación biológica o por ósmosis inversa. Durante el uso de 2-propanol en productos de consumo se producen emisiones dispersas a la atmósfera.

3. Transporte, distribución y transformación en el medio ambiente

La vía principal de entrada del 2-propanol en el medio ambiente es su emisión a la atmósfera durante la producción, el tratamiento, el almacenamiento, el transporte, el uso y la evacuación. También se producen emisiones al suelo y al agua. Es difícil calcular el volumen que ingresa en cada compartimiento ambiental. No obstante, se calculó que en 1976 la liberación total de este compuesto en la atmósfera fue superior al 50% del 2-propanol producido.

El 2-propanol desaparece rápidamente de la atmósfera por reacción con radicales hidroxilo y arrastrado por la lluvia. A este último proceso se debe el transporte del 2-propanol desde la atmósfera hasta el suelo o el agua. Una vez que está en el suelo, se cree que es muy móvil y que aumenta la permeabilidad del suelo a algunos hidrocarburos aromáticos. El 2-propanol es fácilmente biodegradable, en condiciones tanto aerobias como anaerobias.

La bioacumulación del compuesto no es probable, dados su carácter biodegradable y su miscibilidad total con el agua; su coeficiente de reparto log n-octanol/agua es de 0,14 y su factor de bioconcentración de 0,5.

4. Niveles ambientales y exposición humana

La exposición de la población general se produce por ingestión accidental o intencionada, por la ingestión de alimentos que lo contengan como aromatizante volátil natural o añadido o como residuo de disolvente, y por inhalación durante su uso. Se han encontrado concentraciones de 0,2 a 325 mg por litro en bebidas no alcohólicas y de 50 a 3000 mg por kg en alimentos tras el uso de 2-propanol como disolvente en su producción. La exposición de la

Resumen

población general por inhalación de aire ambiental es baja a causa de su rápida desaparición y degradación. Se han estudiado diversas localizaciones y se han medido concentraciones medias ponderadas en función del tiempo de hasta 35 mg/m^3 en emplazamientos urbanos.

Los trabajadores se ven expuestos al 2-propanol durante la producción del propio compuesto y de acetona y otros derivados, así como durante su uso como disolvente. En la encuesta nacional de exposición ocupacional (1980-83) realizada en los Estados Unidos, se estimó que más de 1,8 millones de trabajadores estaban potencialmente expuestos. En ciertos lugares de trabajo se han medido concentraciones de hasta 1350 mg/m^3, con promedios ponderados en función del tiempo de hasta 500 mg/m^3.

5. Cinética y metabolismo

El 2-propanol se absorbe y distribuye rápidamente por todo el organismo tras su inhalación o ingestión. A dosis elevadas se retrasa la absorción gastrointestinal. Las concentraciones sanguíneas de 2-propanol (detectables cuando se ingiere etanol simultáneamente) o de su metabolito, la acetona, guardan relación con los niveles de exposición. En voluntarios que ingirieron una dosis de 3,75 mg/kg (con 1200 mg de etanol/kg) en zumo de naranja, se observó un nivel máximo de 0,8 ± 0,3 mg de 2-propanol libre por litro en la sangre, y de 2,3 ± 1,4 mg por litro tras la incubación con arilsulfatasa, lo que es un signo de sulfatación. Los trabajadores expuestos a vapores (8–647 mg/m^3) mostraron concentraciones de 3–270 mg/m^3 en el aire alveolar, pero en este caso se encontró acetona y no 2-propanol en la sangre y la orina. En animales de laboratorio tratados, el 2-propanol se detectó no sólo en la sangre sino también en el líquido espinal, el hígado, los riñones y el cerebro. Atraviesa la barrera hematocerebral dos veces mejor que el etanol. El 2-propanol se excreta en parte como tal y en parte como acetona, principalmente por vía pulmonar, pero también en la saliva y el jugo gástrico. La reabsorción puede producirse después de la excreción por las últimas dos vías. La transformación en acetona por medio de la deshidrogenasa alcohólica del hígado es más bien lenta, porque la afinidad relativa de la deshidrogenasa por el 2-propanol es más baja que por el etanol. *In vitro*, la actividad enzimática de la deshidrogenasa humana con 2-propanol fue del 9–10% de la actividad que exhibe cuando el sustrato es el etanol. *In vitro* las oxidasas microsómicas de hígado de rata también son capaces de oxidar el 2-propanol. En el hombre, la acetona se excreta sin cambios, principalmente por los pulmones y en cantidad mínima por los riñones. La concentración de acetona en el aire alveolar, la sangre y la orina aumenta con la intensidad y la duración de la exposición al 2-propanol. La eliminación de 2-propanol y de acetona del organismo es de primer orden, y los periodos de semieliminación en el hombre son de 2,5–6,4 horas y 22 horas, respectivamente.

6. Efectos en los organismos en el medio ambiente

La toxicidad del 2-propanol para organismos acuáticos, insectos y plantas es baja. El umbral inhibitorio para la multiplicación celular de una especie de protozoo sensible varió de 104 a 4930 mg por litro en diversas condiciones experimentales. Avanzando en la cadena filogenética, varias especies de crustáceos, incluida *Daphnia magna*, mostraron CE_{50} a concentraciones que iban desde 2285 hasta 9714 mg por litro. Las CL_{50} (96 h) para peces de agua dulce variaron desde 4200 hasta 11 130 mg por litro. Los datos obtenidos para especies de moscas de la fruta mostraron CL_{50} comprendidas entre 10 200 y 13 340 mg por litro de medio nutritivo. La CL_{50} para larvas de mosquito (*Aedes aegypti*) en la tercera etapa de desarrollo fue de 25–120 mg/litro en un ensayo estático de 4 horas.

Los efectos que tiene en las plantas la exposición a 2-propanol en concentraciones entre 2100 mg/litro y más de 36 000 mg/litro variaron entre la ausencia de efecto y la inhibición total de la germinación.

7. Efectos en animales de experimentación y en sistemas de ensayo *in vitro*

La toxicidad aguda del 2-propanol para los mamíferos, a juzgar por la mortalidad, es baja, sea cual sea la vía de exposición oral, cutánea o respiratoria. Los valores de la DL_{50} para varias especies animales tras la administración oral variaron entre 4475 y 7990 mg por kg de peso corporal; La CL_{50} de inhalación durante 8 horas en la rata varió de 46 000 a 55 000 mg por m^3 de aire. A estos niveles letales, las ratas mostraron grave irritación de las mucosas y depresión profunda del sistema nervioso central. La muerte fue provocada por paro respiratorio o cardiaco. Entre las lesiones histopatológicas figuraron la congestión y el edema pulmonar, así como la degeneración celular en el hígado.

Con dosis orales únicas de 3000 ó 6000 mg de 2-propanol por kg de peso corporal se produjo una acumulación reversible de triglicéridos en el hígado de la rata. En la rata se observó inducción de enzimas microsómicas a dosis orales de 390 mg/kg.

El 2-propanol sin diluir no produjo irritaciones cuando se aplicó a la piel cortada o raspada del conejo durante 4 horas. En cambio, se observó irritación cuando se aplicó 0,1 ml de compuesto sin diluir en el ojo del conejo. Con concentraciones de vapor elevadas de 2-propanol se produjo irritación del tracto respiratorio en el ratón, y el ritmo respiratorio disminuyó en un 50% a concentraciones de 12 300–43 525 mg/m^3 de aire.

Se han hecho escasos estudios de exposición repetida sobre los efectos del 2-propanol en animales. Tras la inhalación de 500 mg de 2-propanol/m^3 durante 5 días a la semana y 4 horas al día durante más de 4 meses, se observaron irritación del tracto respiratorio, cambios hematológicos y alteraciones histopatológicas en el hígado y el bazo de la rata. En otro grupo de estudio, se administró a 5 ratas de cada sexo agua de bebida que contenía 2-propanol durante 27 semanas. La comparación de animales que recibían aproximadamente 600 ó 2300 mg por kg al día (machos) y 1000 ó 3900 mg por kg al día (hembras) con grupos de control no tratados reveló un retraso del crecimiento sólo en ambos grupos de hembras expuestas. No se observaron otros efectos adversos.

Los datos disponibles indican que los efectos del 2-propanol en el sistema nervioso central son semejantes a los del etanol. La DE$_{50}$ por vía oral para la narcosis en conejos es de 2280 mg/kg; la DE$_{50}$ intraperitoneal correspondiente a la pérdida del reflejo de enderezamiento en el ratón es de 165 mg/kg, y el umbral intraperitoneal de inducción de ataxia en la rata es de 1106 mg/kg. Estos valores son aproximadamente dos veces más bajos que los correspondientes al etanol. La inhalación de 2-propanol a una concentración de 739 mg/m^3 durante 6 horas al día y 5 días a la semana durante 15 semanas no originó ningún resultado adverso en un ensayo en campo abierto.

El 2-propanol se evaluó en un estudio de 2 generaciones de ratas mediante la administración de 1290, 1380 ó 1470 mg por kg al día en el agua de bebida a ambas generaciones. El único efecto adverso observado fue una reducción transitoria del ritmo de crecimiento en la generación F_0. En cambio, otros investigadores observaron un aumento de las malformaciones en un estudio de la teratogénesis después de administrar por vía oral a ratas gestantes 252 ó 1008 mg de 2-propanol por kg al día (no se formularon observaciones sobre la toxicidad materna). Ambas dosis, administradas en el agua de bebida durante 45 días, también aumentaron la duración del ciclo estrual hasta 5 días (frente a 4 días en los sujetos de control). Se observó una mortalidad embrionaria total mayor cuando se administraban a la rata hembra dosis de 1800 mg/kg en el agua de bebida al día durante 6 meses antes de criar; se notificaron diversos efectos en la supervivencia intrauterina y puerperal a dosis tan bajas como 0,18 mg/kg al día, pero no se observó ninguna pauta coherente. Se expusieron ratas gestantes a 2-propanol atmosférico a concentraciones de 9001, 18 327 ó 23 210 mg por m^3 (3659, 7450 ó 9435 ppm). Las dos concentraciones más elevadas fueron tóxicas para las madres, pero no así la de 9001 mg/m^3. Se observó toxicidad en el desarrollo con las tres concentraciones.

El 2-propanol dio resultados negativos en una prueba con 0,18 mg por placa para detectar mutuaciones puntuales en *S. typhimurium* y en una prueba de intercambio de cromátidas hermanas en fibroblastos pulmonares de hámster chino. Indujo anomalías mitóticas en células de médula ósea de rata y en células de ápice radicular de cebolla *in vitro*. No se dispone de otros datos sobre mutagenicidad.

El 2-propanol se ensayó en varios estudios limitados de carcinogenicidad en el ratón utilizando las vías de exposición cutánea (3 veces a la semana durante un año), inhalación (7700 mg/m^3 durante 3–7 h/día, 5 días/semana, durante 5-8 meses) y subcutánea (20 mg sin diluir, semanalmente durante 20-40 semanas). La aparición de tumores se investigó en los tres estudios en la piel, el pulmón y el lugar de inyección, respectivamente. No se observaron efectos carcinogénicos. No se dispone de datos epidemiológicos adecuados con los que evaluar la carcinogenicidad del 2-propanol para el ser humano. Los datos disponibles indican que el di-2-propilsulfato, un producto intermedio en los procesos de ácidos fuertes y débiles para producir 2-propanol, puede estar asociado causalmente con la inducción de cáncer del seno paranasal en el ser humano.

8. Efectos en la salud humana

Se han notificado varios casos de intoxicación tras la ingestión oral y también en niños con fiebre a los que se refrescó con esponjas impregnadas con preparaciones con 2-propanol. En casos de envenenamiento, los principales signos son los de la intoxicación alcohólica, en particular náuseas, vómitos, dolores abdominales, gastritis, hipotensión e hipotermia. El 2-propanol deprime el sistema nervioso central unas dos veces más que el etanol, provocando una inconsciencia que termina en coma profundo; puede sobrevenir la muerte por depresión respiratoria. Otros efectos relacionados con el compuesto son la hiperglucemia, elevados niveles de proteínas en el líquido cefalorraquídeo y atelectasia. Aunque se considera que la absorción por la piel es insignificante, en un informe sobre un caso de un niño intoxicado tras refrescársele con una esponja impregnada con 2-propanol, se indicaba que no conviene subestimar el riesgo de absorción dérmica, especialmente en los niños. No se observaron efectos adversos en voluntarios sanos que bebieron diariamente durante 6 semanas un jarabe que contenía 2,6 ó 6,4 mg de 2-propanol/kg. Un grupo de varones voluntarios, cuando se expusieron a vapores de 2-propanol en concentraciones de 490, 980 ó 1970 mg por m^3 de aire durante 3–5 minutos juzgaron que la irritación era "leve" a 980 mg/m^3 y "satisfactoria" para su propia exposición ocupacional de 8 horas.

Las irritaciones de la piel en forma de eritema, quemaduras de segundo y tercer grado y ampollas se notificaron en niños prematuros tras un contacto prolongado con 2-propanol. En ocasiones también se han notificado casos de dermatitis alérgica por contacto.

Se dispone de pocos estudios epidemiológicos sobre mortalidad por cáncer o por otras causas. En un grupo de 71 trabajadores empleados durante más de 5 años en una fábrica de 2-propanol por el proceso del ácido fuerte, se notificaron 7 casos de cáncer, entre ellos 4 de cáncer del seno paranasal. En un estudio de cohortes realizado sobre 779 trabajadores en una fábrica similar, las incidencias reajustadas en función de la edad y del sexo de cáncer del seno y de la laringe fueron 21 veces mayores de lo esperado. El periodo mínimo de latencia fue de 10 años. En otro estudio retrospectivo de cohortes realizado en otra fábrica que utilizaba el proceso del ácido fuerte, había más de 4000 personas-años expuestas. Los resultados mostraron que las tasas de mortalidad por todas las causas y por neoplasmas no eran significativamente mayores de lo previsto. Se llevó a cabo un estudio retrospectivo de cohortes en una planta que fabricaba 2-propanol por el proceso del ácido débil. Había más de 11 000 personas-años expuestas. La tasa de mortalidad debida a todas las causas fue más baja de lo esperado. No se observó mortalidad excesiva por todos los cánceres. Sin embargo, la incidencia del cáncer de la boca y de la faringe fue 4 veces más elevada de lo previsto. Los estudios de cohortes indican en conjunto un riesgo de cáncer relacionado con el proceso de fabricación con ácido fuerte, pero, en dos pequeños estudios controlados de casos, no se observó correlación alguna entre la exposición a 2-propanol y la incidencia de gliomas o de leucemia linfática.

Algunos informes parecen indicar que la exposición combinada a tetracloruro de carbono y 2-propanol en los trabajadores potencia la toxicidad del primero.

9. Resumen de la evaluación

La exposición del hombre al 2-propanol puede producirse por inhalación durante la fabricación, el tratamiento y el uso tanto ocupacional como doméstico. La exposición a un nivel potencialmente letal en la población general puede producirse por ingestión accidental o intencionada y los niños pueden estar expuestos cuando se les refresca con esponjas impregnadas con preparaciones a base de 2-propanol (alcohol para friegas).

El 2-propanol se absorbe y distribuye rápidamente por todo el organismo, en parte en forma de acetona. Los datos sobre exposición-efecto en el hombre en condiciones de sobreexposición aguda son escasos y muestran grandes variaciones. Los principales efectos son la gastritis, la depresión del sistema nervioso central con hipotermia y depresión respiratoria, y la hipotensión. Los datos de mortalidad aguda en animales de experimentación indican que la toxicidad del 2-propanol es baja, siendo los valores de DL_{50} orales en diversas especies entre 4475 y 7990 mg/kg, y los valores de CL_{50} de inhalación en ratas alrededor de 50 000 mg/m^3. En el conejo, el 2-propanol no produjo irritaciones cutáneas, pero la aplicación de 0,1 ml de 2-propanol sin diluir produjo irritación en los ojos.

En el hombre, los efectos agudos más probables de la exposición a concentraciones elevadas de 2-propanol por ingestión o inhalación son la intoxicación alcohólica y la narcosis.

No se han hecho suficientes estudios en animales como para evaluar los riesgos que entraña para la salud humana la exposición repetida al 2-propanol. No obstante, los resultados de dos estudios a corto plazo en la rata, incluida la exposición por inhalación (500 mg/m^3 durante 4 horas al día y 5 días a la semana durante 4 meses) y la exposición oral (600–3900 mg/kg en el agua de bebida) indican que debe evitarse la exposición al 2-propanol en algunos de los muy elevados niveles de exposición ocupacional que se han notificado.

La exposición por inhalación de ratas gestantes a 2-propanol dio un nivel mínimo de observación de efectos de 18 327 mg/m^3 (7450 ppm) y un nivel sin efectos observados de 9001 mg/m^3 (3659 ppm) respecto a la toxicidad materna. En el mismo estudio, 9001 mg/m^3 (3659 ppm) fue el nivel más bajo de observación de efectos en lo que respecta a la toxicidad de desarrollo; no se indicó nivel sin efectos observados. Estas concentraciones son más elevadas que las que normalmente se registran en condiciones de exposición humana.

El 2-propanol dio resultado negativo en las pruebas de genotoxicidad, pero indujo aberraciones mitóticas en la médula ósea de la rata. Aunque estos resultados indican que la sustancia no tiene potencial genotóxico, no puede hacerse una evaluación correcta de la mutagenicidad basándose en datos tan limitados.

Los datos disponibles no bastan para evaluar la carcinogenicidad del 2-propanol en animales de experimentación. No se dispone de datos para evaluar la carcinogenicidad del 2-propanol en el ser humano.

Es poco probable que el 2-propanol plantee un riesgo grave para la salud de la población general en las condiciones de exposición que se producen normalmente.

El 2-propanol desaparece rápidamente (periodo de semieliminación 2,5 días) de la atmósfera y su desaparición del agua y del suelo se produce rápidamente por biodegradación aerobia y anaerobia, especialmente tras la adaptación de microorganismos inicialmente sembrados. En vista de las propiedades físicas del 2-propanol, su potencial de bioacumulación es bajo. No representa un riesgo para los organismos naturales en las concentraciones en que suele encontrarse en el medio ambiente.

www.ingramcontent.com/pod-product-compliance
Ingram Content Group UK Ltd.
Pitfield, Milton Keynes, MK11 3LW, UK
UKHW021310180426
11947UKWH00015B/1141